# ADDENDUM

1. On page 223 under the section of Useful Addresses please note an error. The e-mail address of Miccant is miccant@miccant.com.

2. All repertorisations are taken from Isis and reproduced with the kind permission of Miccant Ltd.

# WHAT ABOUT THE POTENCY?

(a comprehensive guide to
homeopathic potency and
dosage)

## BY

## Michelle Shine

FOOD FOR THOUGHT PUBLICATIONS

Food For Thought Publications
Room 6, Concorde House,
Grenville Place,
London NW7 3SA.

Published by Food For Thought Publications
2004

ISBN 0-9547033-0-8

Printed and bound in Great Britain by Biddles Ltd, King's Lynn, Norfolk

Book design by Ruth Kaye

# FOREWORD

This ambitious book shines a light on a relatively neglected area of homeopathic methodology – potency. It provides a beautiful opportunity to peruse this fascinating subject at length, to immerse oneself in a long and thoughtful conversation about potency, for that is how this lovely book is offered – as a discussion based on many years of one homeopath's clinical experience. The subject ripples out into a larger homeopathic pool with interviews with well respected homeopaths who share their insights and experience.

We are a community that loves books – that loves to write, one that has been writing abundantly for nearly two hundred years. It is strange then, that we don't have any books dedicated to potency. This brave book is the first on the subject and it is both frank and pragmatic. How generous of Michelle Shine to allow us such an extensive look into the workings of her mind and her practice.

I wish I had had this book when I started out on my homeopathic journeys in the early 1980s, stumbling over potency and even falling flat on my face at times. My teacher was a fearless prescriber, giving 10Ms – often a different 10M – at every visit. I remember giving Phosphorus 10M to a patient with irritable bowel syndrome, migraines, depression and chronic fatigue amongst many other symptoms. I gave a 10M because I was confident in my remedy – it fit his totality of symptoms including keynotes in every area, aetiology, and mental and emotional symptoms. I gave a 10M because I had inherited a certain fearlessness from my teacher. My patient had a horrible aggravation. For over a month he suffered a great deal. OK, so he was cured, but at what price? I felt terrible - terrible about learning the hard way to first do no harm.

3

I remember studying with many fine teachers, learning many different methods over the years. Learning to start with a 200c from the Greeks, from George Vithoulkas and Vassilis Ghegas, and 'topping it up' with a 6c or 12c – or using the lower potencies to mitigate the worst effects of an aggravation. In the end there were too many aggravations for me to be entirely happy with this method.

I learnt to repeat low potencies from Francisco Eizyaga – stepping up three centesimal doses at a time. Instead of leaping from 6c to 30c, going to 9c and then 12c and so on. This was quite remarkable with deep seated, long term, chronic cases. Sensitive patients were vulnerable to developing proving symptoms rather quickly and needed careful monitoring. I learnt to put a 30c in a dropper bottle and plus it. Patients loved to repeat their remedy and some could not be persuaded to stop on improvement. Again proving symptoms occurred.

I remember learning about the LMs from John Morgan of Helios Pharmacy. I especially remember the confusion and wonder that they brought into my life: finding the rituals of preparation both attractive and a complete drag; finding that two granules instead of one in the stock bottle caused aggravations. Having that literally blow my tiny little mind. I'm sitting here blinking in disbelief as I write this but I know it to be true because I was able to repeat it – both with myself and with a couple of willing patients. It made me wonder about **all** our measurements with **all** of our potencies. It made me wonder a great deal about the **science** of homeopathy.

*What About the Potency?* is full of wonder. There is something on every page – a challenge, a question, a rumination – to encourage the reader to stop and think. This is a rare gift in the written word. I wish I'd had the author's thoughtful reflections to help me in my early years in practice. Michelle Shine's honesty about her own process is a breath of fresh air in a community searching for certainties. It is a bold book – examining doubts and presenting failed cases in equal measure – as well as successes of course. Thank goodness!

The cases along with the deliberations of the prescriber present a riveting gestalt of this homeopath's evolution over time. The author's delightful conversational style makes this a book that is hard to put down. *What About the Potency?* leaves virtually no potency stone unturned. It is a must-read for every student dazed or confused by the whole subject, as well as any practitioner who wants a springboard for reflecting on their own process with potency.

Miranda Castro FSHom, Fort Lauderdale, Florida – October 2004

**To know the unknown, one has to know the known properly.**

B.K.S. Iyengar

Astadala Yogamala – Vol 2

**Do not seek to follow in the footsteps of the men of old; seek what they sought.**

Matsuo Basho, Japanese Poet

FOR ALL MY PATIENTS,
WITHOUT WHOM
THIS BOOK COULD NEVER
HAVE BEEN WRITTEN.

# CONTENTS

## PART ONE

# PART TWO
# THE INTERVIEWS

# INTRODUCTION

I would like to share with you my inspiration for writing this book. I have been in practice now for almost ten years and it has been my good fortune to have built up a very busy practice. I see between twenty and thirty patients a week, and together with looking after my family, (three children, husband, cat, hamster and home), it has been a challenge for me to find space to devote to this project.

Experience is a wonderful teacher. Experience together with the guidance of other long standing and enlightened homeopaths has taught me how to sharpen my case taking skills, to understand the information I have collected, and most importantly, how to find an appropriate remedy.

I feel I have, very quietly, just arrived in a comfortable place, where I can say that I am a competent homeopath and health practitioner.

Advice on potency, however, has been difficult to come by, and my experience on the subject has required a lot of meditation in order to arrive at a workable level of knowledge and understanding.

In the past, often feeling intellectually unequipped, I would resort to dowsing for a choice of potency, and although this method proved to be fairly efficient, it left me ignorant of the understanding that I craved.

Please do not get me wrong. Do not think that at this juncture I purport to have found the last word on the subject. On the contrary, although my explorations have taken me further down the road of discovery, there is still a whole universe of knowledge yet to be claimed.

It is for this reason that I have divided this work into two parts. The first half refers to my professional experiences and conclusions about potency and dosage. The second part is a series of interviews with ten amazing homeopaths, who all work in different ways due to their independent findings and conclusions.

My desire, therefore, is to bring this area of homeopathy to the table, and in doing so, report some interesting and valuable information. This was my inspiration, and I hope that you, the reader, will find the use of this book like a helping hand, lightening the load along the path of your chosen career.

# SOMEWHERE ALONG THE ROAD OF DISCOVERY.....

# WHAT IS HOMEOPATHIC POTENCY?

Of course every homeopath knows that a remedy does not become homeopathic until it is prescribed according to the law of similars.  But what about potency?  In effect every substance that has been diluted and succussed is a remedy in a potency.  The potency is determined by how much the substance has been diluted and how many times succussed.

As it is beyond the scope of this book to give pharmaceutical advice, I would refer the reader to the Organon, aphorism 270, where Samuel Hahnemann gives detailed advice about how to change a crude substance into a dynamic medicine with a potency ascribed.

The idea is to match not only the remedy to the patient or problem, but also the potency should fit with the energy of the problem or with the energy of the vital force.

I think many homeopaths would agree that higher energy should be mirrored with a higher potency. Low energy should be mirrored with a lower potency (SEE CHAPTER ON ENERGY page 109).

# DOES POTENCY REALLY MATTER?

When I left The College of Homeopathy in 1993, I concluded that it was far more important to find a curative remedy than an accurate potency. I remember as a student how every case presented by my lecturers was met by a hand in the air of some eager young hopeful, desperate to be enlightened about potency. 'What potency did you use?' was the most regularly posed question throughout my training, and one that was either waved away with a glib, 'don't worry about that' or answered off-handedly before moving on to, what was in their view a more pressing topic.

Consequently, I determined that potency really did not matter much at all. Then came the stories about how so-and-so prescribed *Sulphur* 10M for an eczema case and how that patient ended up in hospital with a severe aggravation, and suddenly potency did matter. It mattered a lot. Eczema became the dreaded pathology amongst my peers. Everyone was frightened. The advice that was given to us at the time was never to prescribe a high potency for eczema, and things will be okay; but still we were anxious.

Homeopathy had suddenly been transported in our minds from a gentle curative medicine into something that had the potential for making a sick person sicker. It raised my concerns. Suppose that all I can do in certain circumstances is to prescribe something that causes the situation to deteriorate and then have to sit back and watch whilst my patient gets carried away on a stretcher? What kind of a profession was I getting myself into? So, as I tried to defend my chosen career at dinner parties amongst a table of sceptics, knee-deep in their incredulity disbelief, I must admit there were times I gulped hard and prayed that what I said and what my instincts told me about the nobleness of homeopathy were in fact true.

I now know that those scary feelings grew out of ignorance. Ignorance about an aspect of homeopathy that has been mostly brushed under the carpet as if it was not important. Therefore, even though we as homeopaths have largely ignored this area of what we do (just try looking for written works on homeopathic potency), we must seek to know more about it, if we are to become better homeopaths with greater prescribing skills.

Homeopaths know that potency is a scientific treasure waiting in the wings for the scientific world to discover and acknowledge, so it stands to reason that there must be a more accurate way to discern an appropriate potency for our patients.   I believe that much of the information we seek to do this with lies inside the subconscious of most of us who have been practising for some years.

My research, therefore, has been a meditation. The joy was talking with other homeopaths, all of whom challenged my understanding so far, in a positive way.


This is my story.

# STARTING OUT

I have been racking my brains to think back on lectures on potency and dosage. My memory tells me that the information we were given at college was very scant. I phoned a girlfriend who qualified alongside me to verify this. She remembers a lecture on LMs where she was told that the more physical the complaint is, the lower the potency you prescribe, and if the case has a mental and emotional factor, this calls for a higher potency. She also remembers another lecturer telling us that in terms of potency, you prescribe whatever you have in stock. And that was pretty much it.

I remember being told that you prescribe high for vital people with a lot of energy, a healthy baby being a good example of this, and low for very old, or very sick people whose vital force does not exhibit much vibrance at all.

It had also been suggested to me that we should be matching the energy of the problem with the energy of the remedy. For example, a high energy state needs a remedy in high potency, and a low energy state needs a low potency. Which means a boil can receive a high potency even in a less energetic person, and a splinter can receive a low potency in a highly energetic person.

I also remember the contradictory example of the above, given by a very charismatic guest speaker at our school, who related an anecdotal case of a young man in a coma who was dying of Aids. He was called by the family to prescribe a remedy for the dying man. He prescribed something in very high potency. On going back to the hospital the next day, his patient was not in his bed, nor was he dead, but in the next room playing pool!

I was confused. There did not seem to be any concrete rules to go by. How was I going to prescribe cautiously (I didn't want to kill anyone) and still get wonderful results?

Why did my son's very deep splinter get expelled from his foot after a single dose of *Silica* 200c, if you need to prescribe low for a physical problem? Why were cautious colleagues of mine prescribing 30c's and treating mental and emotional problems successfully?

To add to this confusion about potency, the warnings issued at college haunted me. You must not prescribe *Natrum muriaticum* for a *Natrum muriaticum* headache, but must prescribe *Bryonia* instead. If you treat someone who smokes cannabis or someone who takes the Pill, forget it, the remedies will not work. Coffee and mint must be avoided by our patients or they will not get better either. What worried me was not the warnings that I had heard, but the ones I had not had the privilege to hear yet. I mean, I might, in my naivety, do some great damage, and that scared me.

I then went along to a post-graduate tutorial and was exposed to the liberating thoughts of Dorothy Wallstein. She advised us to **break all the rules** and find out for ourselves.

For years afterwards, I did exactly that.

# REFLECTING ON THE EARLY YEARS

Looking back on my earliest cases, I notice that I had more success with lower potencies (mostly 6c and 30c). Of course, this could be complete coincidence that I just happened to find a curative remedy every time I gave a low potency, but this is unlikely.

Nowadays I am able to give a high potency remedy and for it to initiate a positive dynamic response within the patient. So, if I analyse the difference between what I brought to my cases then and what I bring to my cases now, I can safely say that four things have changed.

Firstly, I have more intimate knowledge of many more remedies. Secondly, I am more perceptive. Thirdly, in those days my case taking was always less probing, and finally, I was less self assured. To sum it all up: I was inexperienced.

Even today, when I get the feeling that I am not perceiving something, that my reasons for giving a remedy are shallow, or I am uncertain in any way about my prescription, I will use this internal information as an indication to give a lower potency. (SEE CHAPTER ON SUPERFICIALITY page 28). Here is an example of three of my most successful cases during that early era of my career. Please note that I include them here as examples of low potency prescribing that seemed to work for me.

# CASE ONE
*Female,*
*31 years*


**7.11.95**

*Presenting:* endometriosis diagnosed in 1991.

*Symptoms:* pulling sensation in lower abdomen on movement, feels as if something would rip < on standing and walking> pressure, a tearing pain.

Had a laparoscopy which revealed cysts in ovaries.

Stomach rumbles and is bloated < leading up to menses, during and after.

Can't stand for long periods and sometimes can feel pain when sitting.

Has IBS: constipation alternating with diarrhoea, can be blood in both types of stool and these symptoms are worse around menstruation.

It hurts to pass water around menstruation.

Facial skin was fine until went on the Pill and has got worse since the endometriosis. Now has acne cysts on chin, nose and all over her body, especially on bottom and thighs.

Since diagnosed with endometriosis she has put on four stone.

Period is very heavy with large clots and lasts seven days. Gets moody and aggressive and tearful before and until last day of period.

*Headaches:* has occasional migraine, common type symptoms.

*Indigestion:* can have this even when she doesn't eat. Doctors have said this is from gaining weight. Was put on a male hormone (testosterone, I believe) for a few months which made her breasts smaller and had some positive affect on her acne.

*Appetite:* craves sweet things (3) crisps and dairy (2), averse to spicy or smoked foods.

*Thirst:* has never been a thirsty person.

*Sleep: good.*

*Dreams: losing teeth; feels like something hitting a raw nerve, and someone at the bottom of a cliff.*

*Perspiration: at night can be soaking wet.*

*Fears: worries about keeping in employment and paying the mortgage.*

*Sensitivity: to sun, does not go brown but red, prefers to stay inside in hot weather.*

*Sex: sometimes sex is difficult.*

*Self-description: quite quick-tempered. Lets things get on top of her. Is the first to complain in a restaurant. Not very affectionate. Feels confident when knows what she's doing. Doesn't like to be late or kept waiting.*

*Childhood: was a tomboy. Very sensitive. Was bullied at school. Takes things personally. Used to lie in bed and cry secretly. Doesn't come from an affectionate family. Wasn't brought up to show her feelings. Has barriers. People have to prove themselves to win her trust. Relationships have to be on her terms. Bears grudges.*

**Comment**: *as you can see from the above case, when she talks about her childhood, it suggests Natrum muriaticum to be the constitutional remedy. Yet, Natrum muriaticum people are not usually the first to complain in a restaurant. These days I would have questioned her more around her emotional self to try and understand this discrepancy. I would also question her about her dreams to see how they reflect what's going on in her emotional life. I did not prescribe Natrum muriaticum at the time because my repertorisation suggested a different remedy.*

## Repertorisation:

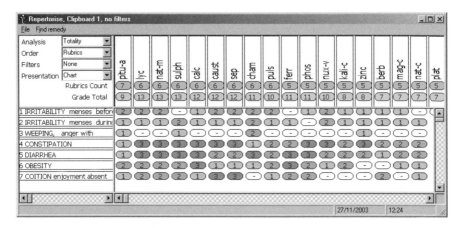

**Analysis:** every one of her symptoms demonstrated that it was her hormonal self that needed fixing. Most of her symptoms were to be found mirrored in the remedy Pituitary anterior, plus it was a remedy that made sense on an organ level too. Interesting that her pains had Bryonia *modalities (the acute of* Natrum muriaticum*).*

**Prescription:** Pituitary anterior 6c bd[1] *diluted and* Bryonia 30c *daily*

## 05.12.95

*Pain better, though still getting odd twinge in lower abdomen*
*Had period with no warning symptoms, lasted 3 days, though heavier than normal.*
*Has started to lose weight.*
*Skin a bit clearer.*
*No IBS symptoms.*
*No pain passing water.*
*No headaches.*
*No indigestion.*
*No craving sweet things*
*Perspiration at night better.*

**Prescription:** *kept her on* Pituitary anterior 6c *and* Bryonia 30c *only when needed.*

---

[1] twice daily.

**17.01.96**

*With period she had minimal amount of pain. Greasy hair and lots of spots came up during period time. Was irritable but only for one day. Had a bit of constipation before her period for a few days.*

*Has taken only two to three doses of Bryonia over the month for the pain. If stands for a long time will get twinges.*

*Everyone is saying how much better she's looking. Eyes bright and face clearer. Stomach has gone down a lot.*

*Spots on body completely gone. Only has spots on her chin at the moment.*

*Had sex for the first time in one and a half years!*

**Comment**: *I did not have access to the proving of Pituitary anterior, nor any other information on the remedy, therefore even though this prescription proved incredibly successful, the remedies were chosen fairly superficially. I gave Pituitary anterior in a 6c with little more indication than a list of symptoms and Bryonia in a 30c because I believed at the time that Bryonia mirrored something a little bit more characteristic and this required a higher potency. It is my belief that this prescription worked so beautifully for three reason: 1. The degree of discomfort from the pathology suggested that prescribing for the disease was the right thing to do. 2. Low potencies were given because of the 'superficiality' of the prescribing. 3. Repeated doses of the remedies were given.*

# CASE TWO
*Male,*
*6 years*


**22.02.94**

*Allopathic diagnosis: ME*

*Mum's description of the problem: up until Christmas very energetic. Since Boxing Day, extremely tired. Very bad, just flopping around. Looked ghostly; white and pale. Didn't want to do anything. Was complaining of pains in his head, both sides. <u>Like in another world.</u> No communication. Doesn't seem to hear others. Still likes reading, but generally can't get it together. Some days he's so slow. Gets bursts of energy, and sometimes he's like his old self. Continuously sucks his thumb. Is sensitive and tearful. Doesn't want to do football training. Used to be Jack the Lad: game for anything. Very popular boy. The leader. Never moans. Falls asleep at 3.20pm on the way home from school. He gets up early, about 5.45 am.*

*His appetite is good. He's allowed one chocolate a day, but he doesn't crave sweets. He likes fish. Doesn't like vegetables. He was very thirsty when he first became ill.*

*Observation: he picks his lips and smiles.*

*Fears: used to fear fireworks and thunderstorms.*

*He never loses his temper. He's well balanced and not moody.*

*He likes music and sings and wants to play an instrument. He dances and pretends he's Michael Jackson. But right now, mum feels he's just going through the motions. He likes cuddles. If criticised he gets upset and goes up to his bedroom and sleeps.*

*He has three red circles on his leg that itch and appear worse after bathing.*

**Repertorisation:**

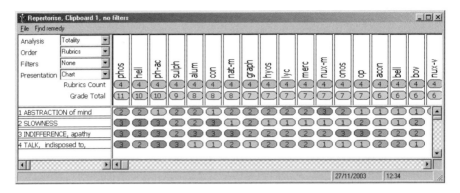

**Prescription**: Nux moschata 30c, split dose.


## 22.03.94

*Much better. Steady progression of getting better. Energy better. He's lasting through the day now. Concentration is better. Skin colour better. The marks on his legs have disappeared. He's playing with his friends again. No spaciness. No slowness. Still slightly sensitive but getting better. No pains in the head.*


**Comment**: *I think I got lucky with this one. Despite my naive case taking skills, this boy's mum was pretty descriptive and gave a lovely portrait of her son's illness.*

*I decided to give a split dose simply because in those days I did not trust that a single dose would be enough. The potency was decided upon because of the low energy in the case making me wish to prescribe fairly low and the disease picture being fairly well matched making me wish to prescribe higher than a 6c.*

*I am still not sure if it was definitely the simillimum, in fact on reading Boericke, the remedy Helleborus under the Mind section actually states 'Picks lips', as one of the symptoms, and may have been a closer remedy. Constitutionally, he may have been a worn out Phosphorous. Or Phosphoric acid may have been appropriate. Today, I would definitely have probed around for an aetiology and other information surrounding the case. The low potency did work well but would one of the other remedies I mentioned have worked too? Would a higher potency have worked just as well? Would it have aggravated? Would* it have only pointed the way to the simillimum in time by heightening some key symptoms whilst ameliorating others?

Unfortunately, at this moment in time, I am unable to answer any of these questions, but it does occur to me that if we as a profession pool our knowledge on these questions, then through the light of our individual experiences, I am sure we will arrive at some universal truths.

# CASE THREE
*Female*
*32 years*

## 11.10.95

*Presenting: polycystic ovaries. Erratic menstrual period because 'pituitary gland which produces ovarian follicle is not working properly' (patient's words), leading to erratic ovulation.*

*Symptoms: PMS[2] can last all month. Severe constipation. Piles.*
*Doesn't sleep well < lately, lots of stress last two years. Lives on nervous energy.*

*Hormonal problems: always had cramps. Period irregular and heavy. Felt ill when came off the Pill last February. Now has rusty old blood or floods. If period is late gets a headache.*

*Emotionally: weepy and stroppy. Everything upsets her. Ends of her fingers feel like spikes. Has odd dragging pain in groins. Feels as if has no energy. Is like a rag-doll. Wakes unrefreshed. Has totally erratic periods.*

*Always constipated since childhood. Can go once a week or once in three days. Sometimes is uncomfortable. Sometimes OK. Has hard stool, difficult to pass more often than not.*

*Sleep: doesn't need lots of sleep. Only 4-5 hours. Falls asleep OK, then wakes an hour later and dozes. Sleeps on her right hand side, in the foetal position.*

---

[2] Pre-menstrual symptoms

Dreams: dead people.
Standing in Sainsbury's with the Chief Rabbi.
What she will be doing the next day.

Can't do anything. Must keep doing things. Must be running during the day. Feels guilty if does nothing. Is like her dad, the opposite of mum.

Low time of day 5-7 p.m. Always has been even as a child.

Suffers with sinus problems since had second baby. He's five years now. Always been catarrhal. Has post-nasal drip. Had tonsils out when three years old.

Acute hearing. Bad sense of smell.

Gets heartburn < when pre-menstrual. Bread gives her indigestion.

**Comment**: the case goes on and on in this terribly haphazard way. Lots of information, none of it with any depth to it at all.

### Repertorisation:

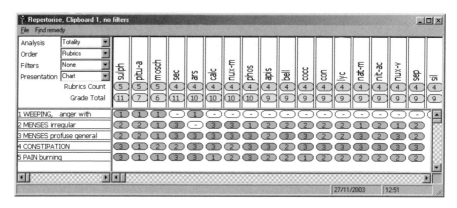

**Prescription:** Pituitary anterior tds[3]

**Comment:** all of her symptoms dramatically improved within a month and within three months the periods and hormonal symptoms were more or less perfect. I saw her again just recently and this improvement has been maintained. My reason for giving this remedy in a low potency is very simple. The fact that most of her PMS symptoms

---

[3] Three times a day

are common symptoms covered by the remedy, and that she had been told that her pituitary gland was not working, made this an indicated remedy on a superficial level. In my understanding superficial equals low potency. The dosage is a standard dosage for a 6c potency.

**Conclusion**: certainly, when it comes to the above three cases, the remedies were close enough to make a huge impact, but were they the simillimum? They might have been, but the answer is inconclusive. What I can say is that, in my experience, **when remedies are given because they seem to mirror the case superficially, then lower potencies seem to work best for my patients.**

# SUPERFICIALITY

All of the three cases so far exhibited in this book have one thing in common and that is a degree of 'superficiality' to the way the remedies were prescribed. That is to say that from my perspective as prescriber, the remedies chosen were superficial to the case.

It could be that the remedy chosen in one or maybe all of the cases was in fact the simillimum, but to the understanding of the prescriber at the time of prescribing, the remedies were 'superficial'. In my own terminology a 'superficial' prescription is based on the following criteria:

- All or many of the symptoms have been exhibited in the remedy given but the character of the remedy is not *seen* exhibited in the patient.
- The prescriber feels he has not understood the case.
- The prescriber has chosen his remedy without being able to distinguish its correctness from another remedy or other remedies.
- The prescriber gets a feeling that the remedy given is not similar enough, probably because the patient's body language is not in keeping with the nature of the remedy given or because the patient's words are not in keeping with his body language upon which the remedy has been chosen, or because the homeopath is not intimate enough with the remedy given.
- The remedy is given because of aetiology, with little other reason.
- The remedy is given because the patient exhibits some keynotes of the remedy given.
- The remedy is given because it is famous for a particular disease i.e. *Lachesis* for menopause.
- The remedy is given because it has an affinity with a particular organ e.g. *Chelidonium* for the liver.
- A nosode is given to address a particular miasmatic taint.

Conversely, and in my own terminology once again, a 'deep' prescription is based on the following reasons:

- The prescriber has understood what needs to be cured in the case and has found a remedy to holistically mirror the patient's dis-ease.

- The prescriber has perceived a strange rare and peculiar symptom that overwhelms the case and he gives the remedy that mirrors this.
- The patient's body language, and his dialogue and the perception of the prescriber all equal the same remedy.
- The remedy given captures the essence of the case.
- The remedy is perceived to have the same characteristic nature as the patient, and therefore one hopes that the remedy will penetrate the depths of the vital force.

# THE CONSTITUTIONAL REMEDY
## versus
# PRESCRIBING FOR THE DISEASE

I have spent an awful lot of years mistakenly thinking that the simillimum is the constitutional remedy. In other words, to be a true homeopath you need to find that ultimate remedy that resonates with the person so completely
they will never need anything else.

These years have not been wasted however. They have taught me to strive to be a better case-taker, to learn more remedies, to hone my skills and endlessly question what I am doing.

After all that, I have come to understand that the constitutional remedy is not always a 'cure all'. Many times, I have given a constitutional remedy and it has not been a 'cure all'. I would imagine that if Francis Treuherz would have received his constitutional remedy and no other treatment instead of *Pyrogen*, he would not be alive today. I also do not believe that treating him with *Pyrogen* at that time was suppression either (SEE FRANCIS TREUHERZ INTERVIEW page 181).

In fact, I think that homeopathic suppression is probably very rare. I cannot remember the last case that I have treated that did not flow in the direction of Hering's Law. If a patient of mine tends to have more resistance to acute ailments, is looking better, and able to cope with their stresses in a better way, if they are more comfortable within their own skin, then I will deduce that they are generally healthier.

In my opinion, the constitutional remedy works best when it is also the remedy for the problem, or to put it another way, when it is the one and only indisputable remedy. As to the potency I would choose in such a situation, see the chapter on higher centesimal potencies.

If the problem has a life of its own and a strong picture aside from the person's normal characteristic self, then you have a choice. You can prescribe either for the problem or for the person. I tend to prescribe upon the picture that overwhelms the case at the time of prescribing.

Frequently I have found that in an acute situation if you prescribe for the person and give the constitutional remedy, you may find that it just will not get there and you will have to prescribe for the problem to resolve the acute circumstance.

However, **prescribing constitutionally or for the disease picture will not in itself influence my choice of potency**.

Here is a case that demonstrates how a very successful constitutional remedy used over a long period of time failed to get to one area of the case, and how another remedy resolved the problem.

## CASE FOUR
*Male*
*5 years*

**21.12.98**

*Presenting: eczema. Hearing problem. Lots of nasal mucus < winter. Complains of headaches and tummy aches.*

*Appetite: fluctuates. Never eats breakfast. If doesn't want to eat makes himself sick. Loves dairy.*

*Early development: his weight is and always has been low.*

*Fears: the dark a little.*

*Personality: quite serious. Quite quiet. Doesn't worry. Gets on well with younger sibling. Likes drawing, watching TV, riding his bicycle, go-karting. Quite tearful recently, mum puts this down to long-term tiredness. Doesn't like making mistakes. Likes to get his own way, cries if he doesn't. Teacher says he is slow to finish his work. He checks to see if what he's heard is correct. He is cautious because he doesn't like to get things wrong. Can be strong willed and stubborn, particularly over food. Will make himself sick if he doesn't want to eat something. Thinks before he does something. He does his work beautifully. Does it just right, even though is pressurised at school to do things faster. He's quite easily led, and can get into trouble for following more dominant and naughty children.*

*Observation: shy. Thinks a long time before answering questions, then whispers to mum.*

**Summary**: *conscientious in his work. Very slim. Lacking in energy. Slowness. Obstinate, but can be yielding too. Desire for milk products. Worse winter.*

**Repertorisation:**

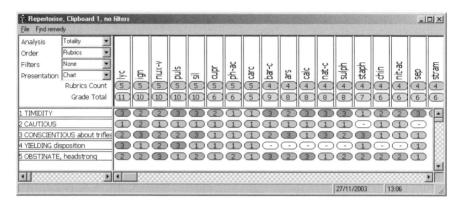

**Prescription**: *Silica LM1, a few drops daily (SEE CHAPTER ON LMs page 49 )*

**Comment:** *At the time of taking this case I was routinely prescribing LM potencies to be administered once daily.*

### 19.01.99

*Hearing vastly improved. Catarrh better. Different in himself, more lively. Eating more and more awake. Eczema better too. Not complaining of headaches and tummy aches so much. Still gets tearful when tired and doesn't want mum to go out in the evenings.*

**Comment**: *basically, he had responded well to Silica since the beginning of his treatment. It had always done a good job whenever his catarrh or hearing problems recurred. I have used Drosera 200c for croup at one stage and Belladonna 30c for a high temperature acute. On 23.03.2001 his mum told me that he gags a lot if he has his top button done up or has a tie on. He doesn't like the toothbrush in his mouth. He also gets hay fever and I have prescribed Silica 200c for that with varying degrees of success (potency chosen because LM wasn't helping and felt a significantly higher potency would be justified in the acute circumstance). Every time I have re-taken his case, it becomes more and more apparent to me that Silica is his constitutional remedy.*

On 26.11.02, I re-took his case by focusing on the symptoms that he had at that time in an acute circumstance.

## 26.11.02

Patient: 'when I cough I feel sick and am worried that I will be sick.'
Mum: 'when he wakes in the morning he feels poorly. Feels sick.'
Observation: he has a sore throat, which is slightly red.

Has a stomach-ache and then needs to go to the toilet. Has runny stools. His chest aches when he coughs. Every night he has had a temperature of 102 degrees in the early evening. Not during the day. Very sweaty at night. No appetite. His sore throat feels like needles and a golf ball.

For the past three months he's been clearing his throat the whole time. He feels as if his throat is blocked up and it makes him want to cough. His voice is croaking.

Mum: 'he's always had a problem with chewing. It's as if he's frightened of swallowing. Strong gagging reflex. I only have to wave a toothbrush and he gags. He fears choking and has done since a baby.'

Patient: ' it feels like I don't want to do it. I don't like gagging. Doesn't feel nice when something hits the back of my mouth.'

Mum: 'he panics and spits things out. He was worried on Friday about his exams. He panicked when he saw a paper. He panics, cries, feels he won't write anything. He sets himself targets. Says,'I can't do this. I've failed'. He had nightmares last week, he didn't want to be alone, woke up in a panic. Last week needed to draw a big circle with his arms. He feels better moving around outside in the garden and kicking a ball.'

**Analysis**: all of this information points to the Cactus plant family which characteristically has a sensation of constriction and a reaction of trying to become bigger or needing to expand (see Sankaran's book An Insight Into Plants). Miasmatically, he was expressing the acute miasm which represents as panic. The remedy of this plant family together with the acute miasm was unobtainable. I therefore gave him another remedy that was obtainable from this plant family. I gave him the remedy appertaining to the typhoid miasm, which according *to Sankaran also has acute episodes, and I hoped the remedy would be close enough to get the desired reaction.*

**Prescription**: Carnegia gigantia 1M daily for 3 days.

### Analysis Demonstration Using Isis:

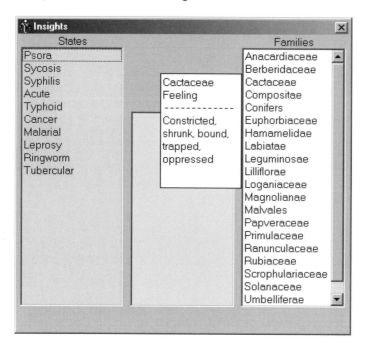

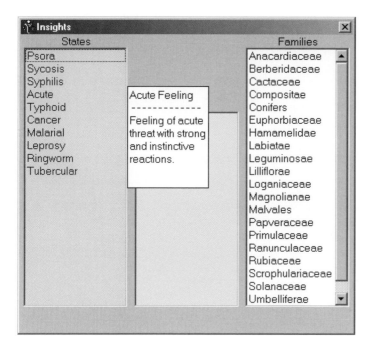

**Comment:** *I chose the potency simply because it was what I had in stock at the time and also because I thought the remedy mirrored the complaint well enough to warrant a high potency. The dosage was a standard dosage that I often give with a 1M.*

### 17.02.03

*Huge, almost instantaneous improvement, for his cough. Now he is not so fazed by eating. Still gets constriction in his throat a little bit, but nowhere near as much as before. Sometimes when nervous gets a lump in his throat, otherwise no...*

**Comment:** *the problem with gagging in his throat had been there since we first met, and although the constitutional remedy helped him enormously, and improved his constitution generally, it also slowly and over the years helped to highlight a specific remedy to deal with this problem.*

*And here is a case that is interesting in terms of both potency and how the case panned out in the follow-up consultation.*

# CASE FIVE
*Female*
*33 years*

*Presenting: a mystery virus, had for 7 weeks*

*Symptoms: swelling in joints of fingers and knees*
*elbows and shoulders. Like a bad inflammation.*
*Pains wandering from one joint to the next. Lethargic.*
*going to bed at 9pm. In the evening whole body stiffens up*
*and can't walk. A hot bath helps (Rhus-tox). Sleepless from pain.*
*Feels very cold. Even when in Dubai had to go back to*
*the hotel and have hot baths.*

*Story: three years ago had lots of tragedy. Husband left her and mum*
*died 2 weeks later. Met someone 8 weeks ago and then got really ill.*
*'I didn't deal with mum's death really well. I blanked it out. I also*
*changed my career. I got made redundant last year. Now I am a self-*
*employed singing teacher.'*

*'Since I met this new chap, I've had very bad insecurities. I'm just*
*waiting to be dumped. I was totally confident and calm before.'*

*Fears: being on her own. 'I've only got dad left and I worry about*
*what's going to happen to him.'*

*Fears: failure.*

*'I take Minocin for acne. When mum died I had a very bad attack.'*
*Also had bad acne when wasn't getting the work in show business that*
*she was trying to break into, and at that time her husband was away a*
*lot too.*

*Growing up: Idyllic. The only child. Very loved by both parents. Too*
*cosseted by mum. 'Miss Goody Two Shoes'. Wouldn't say boo to a*
*goose. Was very clingy to parents, especially mum.*

*Adolesence: 'Miss Goody Two Shoes again'. Sailed right through it.*
*Was stressed when studying singing. Didn't sing well. Also felt was too*
*tall, and then came the spots.*

*Confidence:* to a certain extent. Puts on a confident exterior. Not underneath. Underneath is a shy person. Would really like to sit in a corner and hide away. Must push self to have a personality, and lots of people say she has a good personality. 'Mum pushed me to sing. She wanted me to do well with that. I might not have gone in that direction if she hadn't. Would have done something more low profile.' Anticipatory, and also with new men comes over more confident than she feels.

*Worst thing:* 'Mum dying. I was devastated when my husband left. Mum supported me through that difficult time. Mum was a huge part of my life. Almost unnatural relationship. I was close to mum. She had a lot of say in my life. If I went out I would have to phone her to say I was safe.'

*Self-description:* 'Very tactile, and this new guy is not, and I take that as a rejection. I have to back off. I would be all over someone like a leech. I'm quite a warm, generous person and I like to buy gifts for friends. I have huge worries, even if a person looks at me funny. I think, 'Oh, I've really upset them.' I used to think that it's because I'm a singer that mum loves me. Mum never wanted to hear that I didn't want to do it. I get my moods from other people's moods. I've got a failure complex. I fear failure. I've got lots and lots of love to give.'

*To live with:* 'Fairly easy going. I fall into the wife role very easily. I'm tidy, not obsessively.

### Repertorisation:

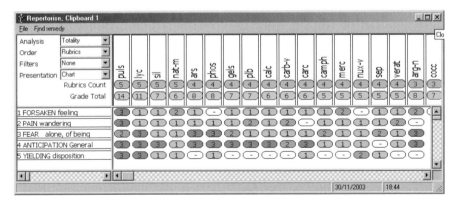

**Comment:** *Clingy, yielding, wandering pains; is there any mistaking the remedy as* Pulsatilla?

***Prescription****:*  Pulsatilla *LM1*

## Phone call 22.11.00

*Main complaint got better after a few days and is now worse again.*

***Advice****:*  *Stop remedy and phone in a few days.*

## Phone call 24.11.00

*No change since 22.11.00.*

***Prescription:*** Pulsatilla *10M csd*

***Comment:***  *I am not sure why I gave an LM to start off with.  I can only say in retrospect that it did not prove to be the best potency.  When things got worse again after an initial improvement, I immediately thought that perhaps it was the result of too much repetition of the remedy in such a short space of time.  With this in mind, I took her off the remedy, but after a few days when the healing process had not continued, I decided that drastic measures were called for.  At that point in time, the remedy was not in question.  I was more than sure of my choice of remedy.  This suggested to me that a much higher potency was necessary, and that is why I gave a 10M.*

### 02.12.00

*Slight pain in knees.*
*Over the weekend had slight pain in shoulders and hands.*
*Now, feels like she's almost back to normal.*
*Cold feeling is gone.  Appetite better now.*
*Feels a lot better in self.  But there is something she has forgotten to tell me.  Since having all the pains she hasn't been able to sing well.  Her voice keeps cutting out.  When mother died couldn't sing for a year.  Is so worried that her joint pains had an affect on her voice. ' I'm such a negative person, no-one will want me now'.*

***Comment:***  *Please read Rajan Sankaran's description of Argentum metallicum, and see if it does not give a beautiful description of this case. In* The Spirit of Homeopathy, *Rajan says 'The situational materia* *medica of Argentum metallicum is that he has been forced by his parents to perform, to be a performer... The parent expects the child to show the world how talented he is and the child feels this as the condition of acceptance by his parents'. Did she not say in the first consultation that she believes it is because she is a singer that her mum loved her? Loss of voice for singers and performers is a keynote of this remedy. She also has a fear of failure, which is a keynote of Argentum nitricum). In this case we must ask ourselves why is she afraid of failure? Answer: because success equals love.*

*I could have waited, but I decided to give this remedy. Ordinarily, I would have given a higher potency with such a clear indication, but because I had just given Pulsatilla 10M, in this case I felt like I wanted to mirror the picture but also complement the previous remedy and not totally overwhelm the vital force with it. It might be illogical, and I cannot substantiate it with this case, but it was my feeling that if I gave a lower potency that this would happen.*

**Prescription**: *Argentum metallicum 200c , one dose split over consecutive nights.*

**Comment**: *unfortunately, I lost touch with her then, and don't know what happened. Once again, I was very sure of the remedy and in retrospect, I could have gone higher with the Argentum metallicum. It would have been lovely to have had the opportunity to follow this one a bit further.*

*But see how these two remedies followed on, one from the other, in quick succession. The first picture was so vivid and the LM just wasn't high enough. The 10M just cruised right in and did the business. The second remedy picture was always there lurking in the shadows of the case, and the first lesion layer cleared and brought the second layer out.*

A similar thing happened again with the following case, which has one miasmatic situation coming first and another miasmatic layer sitting neatly underneath:

# CASE SIX
*Female*
*35 years*


**18.11.02**

*Feeling low since August. Whole year has been a disaster. Beginning of year had chest infection for two months. 'I have to carry on as normal. I just carry on.'*

*Beginning of August had a bit of a wheeze. Usually uses an inhaler once every eighteen months to two years. Got worse before holidays, and was even worse after, led to Becotide inhaler and didn't get any better. Led to steroids and didn't get any better. Took antibiotics and they didn't work, although felt a bit better after them (very unusual).*

*Went to a specialist and was told that she has two extra ribs. The specialist did some allergy testing which revealed sensitivity to cat hair, dog fur, horse hair, grass, pollen, fungal spores, wheat, cereal, and house dust mites.*

*A couple of weeks ago did a charity fashion show and so started to do sit-ups. Also has a private trainer and dances. In the run up to the fashion show was very fatigued. Took double portions of Echinacea.*

*Feels low, swollen glands, heavy, tired, fatigued. Always has to clear her throat and trying to cough up phlegm. Symptoms are forever changing. On Sunday was doing some climbing with her kids and that led to wheeziness. Never gets to bed before midnight.*

*Juggles her work with kids going to nursery. She feels guilty. 'If I'm at the office, I feel I should be with the kids and if I'm with the kids, I feel I should be at the office. I try to fit everything in. I feel like I'm juggling all of the balls and falling on my head. I always want to do the right thing.' Gets stressed if going to be late, makes her anxious. 'I wouldn't want anyone to do that to me'.*

*Her heart is not in the business anymore. 'I thought I would be a business woman when first had kids. Now, I would just like to be a mum, and be a bit selfish for myself.'*

*Feels trapped. On a conveyor belt. Just wants to catch up.*

*'You'll never find the perfect person to do a job for you.' Has a nanny, but she's 'thick'. Has to spoon-feed her with things to do.*

*Dad: could sleep on the floor. A holocaust survivor. Has papers everywhere.*

*Mum: used to measure between place settings.*

*'I can make a mess and tidy up very quickly afterwards.'*

*'My husband would say that I nag. I'd like him to be tidier. I'll throw his things in the cupboard after four or five days, so that I don't have to see them. I want him to be more interactive with everything. I hardly see him. I won't ask him to change his work. It's frustrating. Husband can work 24 hours a day. I feel sorry for him. I don't like him working on weekends. We rarely have a proper conversation. It's very frustrating.*

*If I had time off would like lie-ins. Long walks outside. Go to the gym. Sort the house out. Learn to cook. Be there for the kids. Prepare puzzles and games.'*

*Worry: 'problems at work, I take them to heart. I think I wish that I wasn't in that position. I like to get things done as quickly as possible.'*

*Growing up: parents were strict. She was very cosseted. Rebelled a bit as a teenager, though never smoked or took drugs.*

*Dream: daughter was drowning.*

*Wouldn't want to stay home generally. Before had kids, used to be out six nights a week and used to wonder where she could go on the seventh night. Loves travelling.*

*Complete chocoholic. If gets addicted to something, can't stop. No self-control.*

*Doesn't like drinking. 'I prefer to be in control.'*

**Summary**: *has a history of TB in her family. Feels trapped and dreams of drowning. Doesn't like restrictions. Has changeable symptoms. Does her work in a hurry in order to try and escape from it. Loves travelling and going out. Physically, her problem is respiratory. Allergies. One of the dreams of a prover of Bacillinum is of a concentration camp, and this lady's father is a holocaust survivor. My understanding of all the above information is that the remedy Tuberculinum is needed.*

**Prescription**: Tuberculinum LM1

## Phone call 4.12.02

*Feels very bad.  Feels as if everything is worse.*

**Prescription**: *Stop remedy and phone in a few days.*


## Phone call 6:12:02

*Feeling much better.*

**Prescription**: *take remedy once every three days.*


**Comment**: *I was fairly sure of the remedy at the time.  I gave an LM because I wanted to build her up and thought at the time that an LM would do that best.  In retrospect, I can see that the repeated doses every day were too much stimulation for her, and therefore one or two doses would have been a better option at first.  Alternatively a few doses of a 200c would probably have worked well too.  A 200c being the centesimal potency of choice because I was fairly sure of the remedy, but her immune system was pretty low and I would therefore not have wished to go much higher.   Once she was feeling a lot better, I did wish to continue the remedy although cautiously.  This was an instinctive decision.  I felt somewhere inside of me that she was going to need more doses of the remedy to carry on with the healing process, because I was viewing the situation as an extended acute.*


## 13.12.02

*Still feels a bit wheezy, it comes and goes.  When went to a friend's house who has three cats, got allergy symptoms 'full throttle'. Wheezing, itchy throat and ears and sneezing.*

*Had a few days after taking the remedy when was on a high, then nose-dived.  After stopping the remedy was well all the time except for a wheeze, but every further dose has aggravated the situation.  Now also has slightly itchy ears.*

*No swollen glands.*
*Tiredness and fatigue is still there.*
*Has green stuff in throat now.  It went, now it has come back.*

*Dreams:  Of martial arts instructor.  Thinks it involved training with him.*

*Thinks if feels better, then will be more positive. Going through a phase where can't be bothered to go to work. Last week stayed at home for a day. Didn't have the energy. Yesterday sorted dad's papers out, which has meant to do for ten years.*

*Wants to escape from going to the office. Trying not to feel guilty when doesn't go to the office. Trying to think 'I am the boss. I don't have to go in when I don't want to'.*

*Thinking of changing days at work. Seeing how can change things around to fit in with current lifestyle.*

*Current stress is children's education. ' Have I done the right thing for my daughter? What can I do for my son? I'm tearing myself apart. All my friends' children are more advanced educationally than mine.' Stomach churned for a few days over these decisions about schools.*

*'Still spoon-feeding nanny, but guy in my office is running things fine.'*

*No inclination to go back to martial arts. Has low blood pressure. Doesn't feel fit enough, though misses it. 'It knocks me.' Feels shattered afterwards. 'Used to give me a high.' Gives inner strength. Feels can do anything. ' Like, I can survive that.'*

*'I don't do things on the spur of the moment. I think very seriously about things. It took two years to get units in living room and make a decision on that. If I know something has a long-term effect, I will take a long time to make a decision. I'm not happy if my house is not a show house. It was when I first got married. In my old life if people came round everything was perfect. If guests come over everything must be 100%. I would like people to think of me as superwoman. I like that description. I'm competent. A good mum, and I want to look young forever. Want to look attractive and feel good about myself and fit.'*

*'Since I saw you last, I haven't used the inhaler at all.'*

**Comment**: *is generally better. Still wheezy, though not using an inhaler now. Some definite shift in where she is currently at. Her main physical problem now is tiredness, and her central focus has changed to concern over doing the right thing. Making the right decision. Wanting to be superwoman. Wanting her house to be a show house. Inherited behaviour from her mother? Interesting, there is cancer on her father's side of the family. The cancer miasm was revealing itself strongly, and I saw this as to be her vital force asking me for another remedy. It was* quite clear to me what she needed right now, but I also got the sense that there were still vital pieces of the jigsaw that were missing, and that I was still learning about her: I felt the picture to be incomplete. I therefore wanted to go fairly high, but not very high.

**Prescription:** Carcinosin 200 daily for three days.

**Comment:** The dosage was a standard one that I was using at that time.

### 04.02.03

Chest complaint has completely disappeared. 'I'm prone to getting sore throats and colds more than I used to. I've got a sore throat at the moment, but no swollen glands.

I can't get myself into bed at a decent time. I've too much to do. I go to bed at midnight and get up at 6.45am.

I don't want to be superwoman. I do too much. Part of the problem is I'd like to retire, and start up again in a few years in a different business. I'm handcuffed to the business. I don't want to upset dad, but I'm not very happy about it. It's a constant annoyance. I have to do the job, but my heart is not in it. Dad says I should let my sister take it over, but she knows nothing about the business and she hates my guts.'

Dream: ' I was on a plane and the pilot said we weren't going to make it. We crashed into the sea and were floating. Next minute we'd lurched forwards and were knee-deep in water. I wasn't scared to die, but scared of pain. Frightened of drowning.'

Is not feeling low.

Phlegm in throat keeps coming and going.

Is still a complete chocoholic.

Still likes order and things done in a certain way. Worked very hard to get house 100% so nanny could see how she likes it kept.

Been getting up earlier because doesn't want to rush.

**Comment**: *much improvement. Still expressing need for order etc, and also feelings of being trapped. This is the second time she has told me about dreams of drowning. When you are drowning, you can't breathe, this is very similar to what happens when someone has an asthma attack. This is her fear. But what to do next seemed unclear and because things were still improving, I decided to wait. In fact, I have seen her recently and she remains well to date, even her sore throats and colds have gone into remission.*

**Conclusion:** I feel that in these situations you give the remedy that is most obvious at the time. If it is the constitutional remedy, it will raise the person's energy enough to a) improve health generally and b) eventually give them enough energy to make obvious the other remedy they need. And sometimes, it will go all the way. Any way you care to look at it, the vital force will lead the way, as a homeopath you only have to follow the signposts that will take your patient to greater health.

Here is a case that went all the way with only one remedy:

# CASE SEVEN
*Female*
*31 years*

**20.11.01**

*Presenting: vaginal infection diagnosed as a beta haemolytic streptococcus with aerobic discharge.*

*Duration: two years.*

*Has a swollen lower abdomen and in the beginning had delayed urination. It presents with a sticky yellow/green discharge in the middle of the month and just after menses. When she stands up feels a pull in her abdomen as if she has stitches. Makes her feel not nice and doesn't want sex. It makes her depressed. Has been trying to fall pregnant again for the past three years.*

*Periods are exactly twenty-eight days, although they can be either early or late. Period lasts between six to eight days. Intermittent period. Is moody and emotional around the time of her period.*

Energy: has a very busy lifestyle. Always running and on the go. Gets to the point when so tired. Finds it difficult to relax. Trying for a child is stressful. Makes her emotional, tearful. In the beginning lost confidence in herself, but as time went by became more accepting and stronger. Gets uptight about things e.g. son's birthday party. Gets indigestion and knots in her stomach after.

Arguments with friends make her stressed. They make her feel insecure. Making dinner parties leads to knots in her stomach. 'Have I got enough time to do it in?'

'If I have a vision in my mind of how I want to do something, it has got to be as I have it in my mind.'

Doesn't scream and shout. It is a calm household. When son was born was very overprotective. Didn't want anyone else to have him, not even her husband. There's only certain people I can trust to have him. Finds it hard to let him go.

'I hardly trust anyone.'

Growing up: ' was wonderful. Very happy house. No arguing. Close to brother. Was nineteen when parents split up. Dad was selfish. He got married again. (Patient very emotional). Family arguments with dad and me in the middle. When I got married, I didn't want to know and shut myself off.' But remains close to mum and resentful of dad...

'I'm very stubborn. I think my way is the right way. I like to have control. If something is not right in my life, I just get rid of it.'

Was babied and cosseted as a child. 'My family never said what they felt.' Never had confidence in talking to new people. In work is a perfectionist. 'Everything has to work out the same way as in my mind. It's important to feel accepted by people. I need to be with people.'

'I like love stories and romance, beautiful things.'

Dreams: Of old house.

'The house I live in now is very similar to the house I grew up in, and I feel very comfortable to sleep in this house. Part of me still feels as if I am a little girl and haven't grown up yet.'

'Once I've done something, that's it. There's no going back. I was very obsessed with a previous boyfriend, and finished with him when my parents split up. I felt insecure with him and didn't trust him. I felt he might finish with me.'

*'I used to daydream a lot at school, about romantic situations.'*

## Repertorisation:

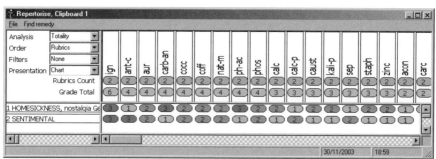

**Prescription:** Antimonium crudum 1M daily for 3 days.

**Summary:** to me, the remedy was very clear. Growing up was wonderful and harmonious. Parents split up and the illusion was shattered. She's sentimental and nostalgic and these days mistrusting. She has high standards even for herself to live up to.

In The Soul of Remedies, Rajan Sankaran says of Antimonium crudum[4], 'In it we see the Antimonium feeling of being let down and disappointed by others, and therefore the need to narrow one's circle, to isolate oneself'. This is expressed in this case by finishing with her boyfriend after her parents split up. Rajan Sankaran goes on to say in his essay of this remedy, 'He (the patient) longs for that which he misses or has been disappointed by: he becomes nostalgic and longs for the past.' In this case I believe that this is mirrored by her dreams, and in my view, the most interesting thing that this patient revealed, which is how the house she lives in now is similar to that of her childhood. She feels comfortable to sleep in this house and that part of her still feels as if she is a little girl not grown up yet.

I needed a remedy that mirrored the essence of her perception. Because the picture was so clear to me I chose a high potency and it worked like a dream. All symptoms cleared up by the next month. By the end of February 2002 the symptoms had returned slightly, and I therefore repeated the remedy. As far as I know, she has remained well to date.

---

[4] *The Soul of Rememdies* by Rajan Sankaran, page 11

# ORGAN SPECIFIC REMEDIES AND TISSUE SALTS

At the other end of the spectrum, or should I say on a more 'superficial' level, there are organ specific remedies and tissue salts. I have had marvellous results with some of these, as have many other homeopaths I have spoken to.

*Calcarea phosphorica* 9x for example, bought because Helios are not able to supply me with the 6x in medicating potency. Two cases that come immediately to mind are:

1. A lady in her early 40s unfortunately suffering from breast cancer and metastasis consulted me because even though she was on HRT her bone density was low and still dropping. After three months on *Calcarea phosphorica* 9x bd her bone density significantly improved.

2. A lady in her 50s not on HRT and worried because her bone density was low was put on *Calcarea phosphorica* 9x bd and within 6 months her bone density had improved dramatically.

I have had similar results with *Calcarea fluorica* 9x for adhesions after operations, and fairly good, but not as consistent, results with *Silica* 9x for weak nails and hair.

I do not tend to use other tissue salts in the same way.

My experiences with a couple of organ specific remedies have been consistently good too.

*Chelidonium* in mother tincture, five drops daily in water or fruit juice for about a week, tends to help out when a patient is feeling nauseous after homeopathic treatment. A symptom which, rightly or wrongly, I diagnose as a sort of detox symptom that indicates a sluggish liver.

*Euphrasia* in mother tincture is almost a perfect specific for conjunctivitis, when used diluted in water to bathe the eye.

Other experiences with either mother tinctures or low potencies have been more random in terms of success.

# EXPERIMENTING WITH LMS

During my final year as a student, I was fortunate to sit in with Peter Chappell. I felt very privileged at the time as he is a very experienced homeopath, and I had come to his practice to complete my shadowing hours and, hopefully, to learn.

One of his prescribing techniques was to almost exclusively prescribe LMs. I remember him telling me that he even prescribed them successfully for acutes. He prepared them differently from the traditional method.

He would drop one granule into (I think it was a 30ml) a dropper bottle, and fill it with mineral water and a drop of alcohol. The patient had instructions to succuss the bottle a number of times and take a few drops on the tongue daily.

Because of my experience with low potencies, and as we were taught LMs were perhaps the lowest and gentlest potency, I began using them.

I prepared them in the same way as Peter Chappell had shown me and I started to use them almost exclusively too. I still always start with an LM1 and move up sequentially when the patient finishes the bottle. I used to ask them to refill it once before moving to the next level, but I found that tiresome and don't do that anymore. I always ask my patients to bang the bottle ten times prior to taking the remedy. Intellectually, it takes the question mark out of what potency I am going to give and makes it easy for me.

I was careful. I would always, at the end of every first consultation, inform my patient as to what to expect from their homeopathic remedy. I would discuss what I was hoping to ultimately achieve by way of the remedy, and I would tell them about aggravations. It was my advice, and still is, that they contact me if they experience anything that they may have previously viewed as negative. It was and still is my policy to stop the remedy immediately if an aggravation occurs. I would often put them back on it again but less frequently; how often being dependent upon their sensitivity.

I have however, had to deal with many aggravations from LMs; a handful of patients who did not come back because they did not like what they were experiencing; a few very horrible skin aggravations; loads that I was able to manage pretty successfully (even some of the horrible skin aggravations) and a few that I could not manage at all, where every subsequent dose aggravated no matter how long the wait in between. For the latter, I would move over to centesimal potencies, and that almost always cured the problem.

What I did learn however, was that if I matched the remedy to the patient/problem correctly, then the majority of patients got well painlessly with a dose of LM repeated every day. Even some eczema cases were cured without aggravating when giving the remedy in this way.

It is a method I use even now, though I tend not to use them quite so often these days. **My gut feeling has been for a while now that the more certain you are of the remedy the higher you go in potency, and therefore, if I'm hesitating, I usually tend to give an LM.**

**If there are maintaining causes, especially if people are on drug therapy, take recreational drugs, or are habitual coffee drinkers, I will give an LM**, though sometimes, you have to get them to give up coffee (especially if the remedy is *Psorinum*). LMs, because of repeated doses, reduce the risk of antidoting and I hate those question-marks: did the remedy run out of steam? How good was the remedy proving to be? Did it get antidoted?

**Some patients like the idea of taking something every day.** *Pulsatillas*, *Arsenicum albums* and *Kali carbonicums*, by their very nature, need to feel constantly supported and **if I get the feeling that a patient needs more support, then psychologically they generally tend to be happier with LMs.** Other patients prefer the idea of a single dose, telling me it's hard for them to remember to take their prescription every day. In these cases, I generally opt for a single or a single collective dose of a centesimal potency.

Here are just a few examples where anLM potency has been successful:

# CASE EIGHT
Male
36 years


**28.01.02**

*Presenting: boils on skin in scalp. 'Getting on my nerves.' Thinks it's linked with extreme stomach cramps when stressed and with anxiety. Thinks it is lifestyle related. Sometimes in morning feels sicks. Feels better after has shaved and had a cup of coffee.*

*Stress: it's my own expectations. I'm an achievement freak. Don't know when to chill or take a step back. 'I have to be top of what I do be aggressive and focused.' I've put myself through a culture shock. I come from nice people and an easy life but contentment doesn't do it. I want to achieve and get on. I've taken on responsibility. Left all family and references behind six years ago when I came to this country. Six years ago I had no responsibility. Had a good job. Was living with parents. It was too easy. It was time to grow up and get on with my life. I worry. I don't feel I have a safety net. I have nothing but myself to fall back on. It is as if I'm not allowed to stop until I have that safety net.'*

*Safety net: financial net*

*'My parents never owned their own home. I have a mortgage. I don't have life long-friends here, my closest family are my in-laws and my wife. My sister lives here, but I don't have a relationship with her. Unconditional love doesn't exist. I have to create that.*

*'I work in a multi-dimensional environment. I don't do one thing at a time. My skills are being analytical. Getting to the bottom of a problem. Understanding causes. Separating what's essential from what is not. There's an element of empathy. Not to pre-judge. Language skills. Reading and writing. Perseverance.'*

*Fears are: 'losing it all. I've seen my father lose it all. It's created an imprint and a stigma on him. I've left it behind. It's been a way to reinvent myself.'*

*Growing up: 'very protected. Come from a small, close knit community. When I left it all, the learning curve was vertical.'*

*Mum: 'very average, neurotic, Jewish mum. Mum left it all behind. She came from Israel. Had ambition for her children. Never worked.'*

Father: ' _Diamond broker_. I have his ambition for me. He told me 'you will not be a diamond broker, you will finish your studies and get the hell out of here.'

Sister: 'Has issues with parents. I disapprove of the way she is towards them. I've come between my parents and sister.'

'When I left Belgium my horizons were average. I had to stand on my own two feet. I have to get myself on the road. I didn't have responsibilities. There's an element of being _excellent at what I do._ There's a taboo about money in my family. An element of guilt. A bizarre relationship to people with money. Mum despises and envies wealthy people, because they're not worthy, not intellectual.'

Excellence is the ability to _juggle all the  elements of his life._

Worries if has to give a talk etc. 'It doesn't impede my functioning. It saps my energy_, cuts me off from people. I lose contact._ I have to think and feel for two (now that he's married). I consider this like being another pressure.

I fly a lot. I'm in a plane. Two pilots and both of them have their energy sapped and the plane goes down (this is another worry for him). I worry about food poisoning. I never eat on a plane.

I'm not schizophrenic. I've become aware when it starts and finishes. It starts in my chest and goes to my abdomen. It feels oppressive and makes me nauseous, and wrapped in a constant _sadness._ It's not pleasant. When I'm in a social situation, I can't enjoy myself. _Don't let people through._' Can't relax fully, almost on the defensive. Feel something bad is going to happen.

Sadness: 'like when someone's dying. You can't go back. It's the end of the road.'

Dream: 'massive row with mother. Woke up feeling what was that all about. _Feeling beside myself._ Must have been angry about something and needed to go and finish it.'

Anger: 'repeated unreasonableness. Irritated at injustice, stupidity, when something could be avoided. Not learning from mistakes. Stubbornness. I'm right. Every one else is wrong. Not achieving something I have decided to, ' swatting a mosquito' syndrome.

To live with: intense. Can be fun. Interesting. Not too untidy. Like refinement around me. Won't buy something because it's a big name.

*I do research things before I buy. I like surrounding myself with music and books. I like to share with people who appreciate these things. I like to have people in my home. Hospitality. To share.*

*'I'm a perfectionist. On a scale of one to ten, I'm eleven.'*

*Depression: 'it's self induced. Some strange, misguided conception. I need at least one thing to go really well. <u>I feel I am very much on my own</u>. Not getting any emotional reward at work. Not satisfied with intellectual stimulation at home.*

*'I've high standards for my wife too. My parents standards are high. Integrity, morality. A lot of my role models are freemasons.'*

## Repertorisation:

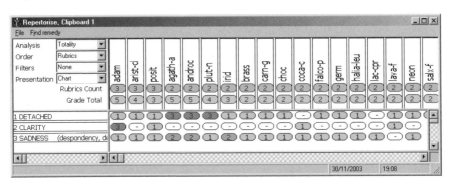

**Comment**: *I have underlined the elements of the case that led me to the remedy. Adamas (Diamond) is a new, recently proved remedy and I had no clinical experience of it to draw upon. Therefore, I really wasn't sure whether to give Aurum metallicum (which was a close fit with its elements of sadness, morality, responsibility and conscientiousness) or Adamas. Anyway, I didn't feel Aurum metallicum was completely right and therefore ultimately decided it had to be Diamond. Because I was unsure of the remedy I gave an LM.*

**Prescription**: *Adamas LM1 daily*

### 04.03.02

*Hasn't had any breakouts of spots.*
*Remedy has reduced stress levels.*
*Drinking more water.*

*Hasn't had any stomach cramps.*
*More careful with what he intakes e.g. red wine.*
*Feeling sick in the morning hasn't occurred.*
*Has sometimes felt a small knot in torso.*
*Still feels doesn't have a 'safety net'.*
*Anxiety not around at the moment*

**Plan**: *carry on with remedy and review in a month.*


## 15.04.02

*No eruptions on scalp.*
*No sickness in the mornings.*
*No  incidents of anxiety.*
*No stomach cramps.*

*Dream: 'Trying to talk to someone and articulate something.  Felt I couldn't speak, like being out of breath.  Felt deprived of the ability to speak as well as out of breath.*

*I still feel suspicious of my self.  Of anxiety attacks coming back, as if I don't trust myself not having them.  Like an addiction.  Sometimes see them coming.  Sometimes it feels good to wallow.  Feels like 'Oh shit, I'm on my own.  I can't rely on anyone else.  I have ultimate responsibility for myself and immediate family. I'm nervous about work.  Under constant scrutiny.  I can't be bothered.  I'm depressed.  Why am I doing this?  I worry; it's the inability to focus and get rid of noise, and I procrastinate.'*

**Plan**: *Stop remedy and speak in two weeks.*


## Phone call 29/04/02.

*Things still in decline.*

**Prescription:** Adamas 1M sd[5]

**Comment**: *I was more sure of the remedy now.  It seemed to be a holistic remedy for him.  When it worked, it wasn't just partially curative. I decided that this potency was no longer high enough to meet his increasing energy levels, even though it was increasing on a daily basis*

---

[5] single dose

by succession, it obviously was not increasing enough. The fact that his decline continued after the remedy was stopped suggested to me that it was from lack of stimulation from a remedy and not over-stimulation which would have eventually gone on to amelioration when not repeated any further. I therefore I decided that a higher potency was appropriate. In a way, I was guessing at what the best potency would be, as my knowledge of this remedy was limited to the proving data and I had no other information to draw upon. A 1M felt right. As far as dosage goes, I was starting to give single doses instead of daily for three days, and in the main it was working well, so I gave a single dose in this instance.

## 27.05.02

Took remedy, and anxiety attacks have not gone.
Had one intense one after receiving the remedy.
Since then panic attacks seem to be becoming less intense.
At the beginning of the month were every two to three days, now every three to four days.
No eruptions on scalp. No sickness in the mornings..
Still feelings of aloneness and 'no safety net'. Thinks 'Who will help me if I'm out of a job?'.

**Prescription**: No remedy at present.

## 01.07.02

Only had a couple of panic attacks and not too intense. But things in scalp have come back. No morning sickness or cramps.
Had feelings of sadness from time to time.

**Comment**: His health seems to be declining a bit again now.

**Prescription:** Adamas 1M daily for three days. (A momentary loss of confidence in the single dose for no reason I can remember).

## 23.09.02

No cramps. No morning sickness. No panic attacks. Things in scalp have gone.
No feelings of sadness.

**Comment**: *doing extremely well.*

**Prescription:** *no remedy necessary.*


### 25.11.02

*Still fine. No instances of anything. Just a dip in energy levels over the last few weeks. Feels flat. 'Everything's a struggle. Everything's difficult.'*


**Comment:** *his vital force seems to have taken a dip in energy once again, and therefore decided to repeat the remedy.*

**Prescription:** *Adamas 1M sd*

**Comment:** *this gentleman is one of the many patients I have treated over the years, in whom it does not seem to matter too much if they have his remedy daily over three days, or just one dose. For some patients I have noticed that three doses over three days is a bit too much stimulation to their vital force and they do express a worsening of symptoms for a short while. This, in my experience, is quite rare.*

# CASE NINE

*Female*
*33 years*

## 11.09.02

Has been on Prozac for three and a half years since daughter was born. If tries to come off it symptoms come straight back.

Got post-natal depression with first and second child that lasted a year both times.

When pregnant with her last (third) child, expected to get depressed.

Feels low if tries to come off Prozac. Gets very uptight with kids, and especially feels that she's not able to cope, almost like a panicky feeling.

Now feels low and irritable even when on Prozac. One week before her period is awful. Wants to be alone, and get out of her situation. Doesn't want to be a mum with kids, the cooking, shopping, or sex with her husband. Energy is flat.

Is quite an organised person and everything has to be just so. 'If I let that go, I'd just feel worse. Would feel totally out of control then.'

Feels better going out with friends, better if exercises…

## Repertorisation:

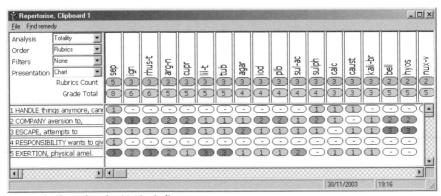

**Prescription:** Sepia LM1 daily

**Comment**: the case goes on, but has nothing more to demonstrate for our purposes here. It is a very clear case of Sepia, and if she hadn't been taking Prozac every day, I would have given a 10M. But because she was on Prozac, I gave Sepia LM1 daily (a standard dosage that I use).

## 07.10.02

A couple of days after seeing me, she ran out of Prozac and decided that she wasn't going to take them anymore.

Had a period just after stopping Prozac and it was awful. Very short fuse. Very tearful, moody. Since then feels more in control. Feels her head is a lot clearer. When on Prozac it feels hazy and fuzzy.

Doesn't feel the need to go back on Prozac. Feels better not on it, and thinks she feels generally better. Still on a short fuse, but hasn't had the feeling that she can't cope.

In the last week, doesn't feel so low. Feels more emotional than low. Very sensitive. Lack of confidence, but doesn't need to be alone so much and her libido is back a bit.
Feels she has a bit more energy...

**Comment**: I kept her on her remedy until 20.01.03. She continued to improve up until that time when she reported that she felt absolutely fine. It is interesting, how in case eight it was necessary for me to ultimately increase the potency, and I chose a fairly high centesimal which got things going again nicely. Yet, in this case, I didn't need to go beyond Sepia LM1.

# CASE TEN
*Female*
*35 years*

**08.07.98**

*Presenting: stomach aches and lots of wind.*

*Takes on lots of responsibilities with her family. Ever since her father died has taken on the role of 'doer'. Doesn't relax easily. If a lot is going on this creates tension in her stomach. Hates flying. Doesn't like to be out of control. Feels sick in boats.*

*A few years ago had very bad and painful wind and would feel sick with acid and burning in her stomach. Sometimes had to lie down with it.*

*Dream: dad didn't really die, but is in hospital still and no-one else knows about it. It was a big secret.*

*Dad died when she was thirteen years old. 'I just accepted it.' I'm the sort of person that just gets on with things. I am bossy, a 'doer'. I would never cry in public. When I first met my husband, he used to call me 'tough-nut'. My grandmother died two weeks after dad. I remember helping out in the house, getting dinner ready. I took on the motherly role.'*

*Fears: cancer and getting ill, because she has the responsibility of the family. If she doesn't take the responsibility, there's no control. Finds it hard to delegate. Never sits down. Is friendly and chatty and kind. 'I'm always helping people out. I plan a lot. Need to be in control. Organised. I do things prematurely. Always plan ahead.'*

## Repertorisation:

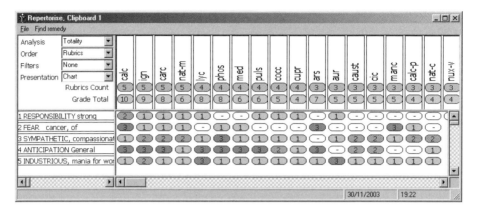

**Prescription:** Carcinosin LM1 daily.

**Comment:** At the time I took this case, it was fairly standard for me to prescribe an LM.

### 28.08.98

For the first week, stomach problems were worse. Now much better. People are commenting that she seems more relaxed lately, and she does feel calmer. 'I don't let things wind me up as much, and feel more positive in general.'

**Comment:** we seemed to clear up the presenting complaint with this prescription, and made her feel better in herself too. She came to see me again two years later when I prescribed Carcinosin LM2 (I very rarely change a remedy that works), and I haven't seen her since.
And here's one that I lost through a not- so-gentle LM:

## CASE ELEVEN

*Female*
*61 years*

*13.09.99*

*Presenting: sleeplessness and depression.*

*Widowed sixteen months ago, and since then sleep has been a problem. Takes Tamazepan. Takes St John's Wort for depression.*

*When gets stressed loses her voice. If exposed to cigarette smoke it leads to coughing the next day. Used to get lower back pain from disc problems. Has metatarsal problems in her feet, 'It's like walking on bone.' When she wakes up in the morning she is nauseous.*

*If she doesn't take Tamazepan she can be wide awake from 2am. Dreamt about her husband last night, and that's the second time since he died. If awake at night then thinks about her husband and aggravation with her children.*

*Gets night sweats.*

*Has lots of energy. <u>Feels very alone</u>. When husband died she went into shock. Finds airports difficult, travelling is difficult. When he was alive, she had never handled money, never paid a bill. Her children are not as supportive as she thinks they should be. She has also been dropped by long-term friends.*

*Her worst time of day is waking. Is desperate to sleep and doesn't want to wake up.*

*'I have no focus, no purpose, no reason. What's it all for?'*

*Her short- term memory is dreadful.*

*Her appetite is very bad. Doesn't eat meat. Doesn't like meat.*

*Has no patience for her grandchildren. Hasn't got the confidence. Feels abandoned by her children. Feels as if this is a major depression. Her eyes are always red and tired and sore and feel as if they are falling out of their sockets.*

*Fears growing old and ending up in a home. Fears falling over and breaking something with no partner to look after her. Fears being* unwell with no-one else there. Fears her mother dying and her brother getting ill. They've both been very supportive.

Her husband kept the whole family together. Patient relied on him for everything. His personality was very big. 'He took away my position.' She had her own problems within the marriage, but was not a good arguer. She doesn't confront. It could lead to another abandonment.

Before her husband died, she was very tidy and clean. Now she sometimes doesn't shower. 'Before he died I was quite off-hand, didn't give people time. I'm more gentle now. I need people now. Much quieter than I used to be. I was buoyant, but now I'm withdrawn.'

'I'm angry about what's happened. I need someone there, not necessarily in the same room. 'I used to be jealous about the relationship that my son had with my husband. I used to be very competitive with golf and bridge. I used to be very up and down, I can be like that now, manic-depressive.'

## Repertorisation:

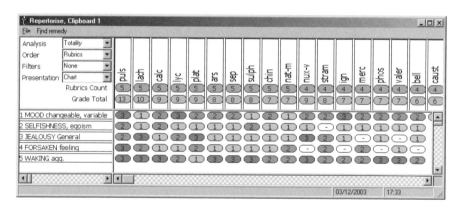

**Prescription:** Lachesis LM1

**Comment**. was this remedy only a partial fit with the competitiveness of the past, the up and downness of her moods, the selfishness and jealousy? Certainly this was no Pulsatilla. I didn't think Ignatia was a good enough remedy either at the time, as she was too needy. However, after Lachesis LM1, her symptoms became much worse and I never had the opportunity to do anything else with her case. I exhibit this case here because I was taught that you cannot get an *aggravation from an LM potency. This case proves that the notion that LMs are too gentle to provoke an aggravation is a fallacy.*

# HIGHER POTENCIES

I will tell you what used to scare me about centesimal potencies: running out of steam too quickly. That was my predominant memory of unrepeated centesimal potencies when I prescribed them in my early years. When this happened, I was not sure what was going on. Was this a good remedy, or just close enough to cause a stir? Has the remedy been antidoted in some way? If so, how can I stop this happening next time? If the remedy runs out of steam after one week and I have seen the patient after four, that means three weeks have been wasted – can the patient/practitioner relationship survive *another* four weeks waiting to find out if this remedy is helpful or not? How long will the patient have faith in me and hang around waiting for me to get it right? Can it be appropriate to give high potencies fairly frequently?

Now, my thoughts around prescribing single dose or split dose centesimals are somewhat more confident. These days when I prescribe in this way they are usually fairly high potencies (ranging from 200c to 50M, depending on the case) and usually do not need repeating a long time before I next see the patient. If they do, I consider changing the remedy, but if I am confident that I have got it right, I will give the remedy as frequently as need be, even if it is a high potency, or I will go up in potency. Generally, they seem to last a good period of time. **I tend to only give them when I get a strong 'gut feeling' that the remedy is a very good one and will not be antidoted, and if in addition the emphasised words of a patient, and their behaviour, tend to indicate that remedy strongly. When the energy of the patient is good (plentiful but not too hyper), I tend to go higher. If the energy is lacking or the patient is hyperactive, I go lower**. Sometimes if the energy is really low or there is lots of pathology, I will give a 6c tds with good results and work my way up through the potencies from there.

I have rarely been disappointed or had aggravations to deal with when prescribing this way. Years of experience have improved my case-taking skills and formed a greater understanding of patients and remedies. When I am less confident about the remedy, I still do better with LMs, or a lower centesimal (6c-30c).

Many of the homeopaths I interviewed agreed with the notion that lack of confidence in the remedy should be matched by a lower potency, and clarity should be matched by a higher potency.

Rajan Sankaran gave the example of an *Opium* case in his book *The System of Homeopathy* where he used, with great results, a 30c potency to begin with because the picture was not exhibited with enough clarity. He comments:

'This was my first case of a remedy belonging to the drug group of addictive substances. This was a whole area I had not understood so far. The only thing I knew about *Opium* was pain/painlessness, visions, constipation. I had nothing better to give him, so I gave him one dose of *Opium* 30c.'

P. Sankaran in his book *The Elements of Homeopathy*, states:

'A patient comes in and says 'I don't know but I often feel that I am poor, that I look like a beggar and am wearing tattered clothes.'

Here we have an intense, clear and spontaneous expression. In such a case, I would almost invariably give a high dose (perhaps a 10M); all other considerations, such as pathology etc., would be secondary.'

# PLUSSING REMEDIES

My first experience of plussing remedies came when I was a student. I had a terrible sinus headache (at least now I presume that is what it was). I remember panicking and calling the doctor, who suggested I go straight to hospital to be tested for meningitis.

Before I left, I called my homeopath and spoke to her locum. The locum requested I dissolve an Arsenicum 200c in a half a glass of still mineral water, stir the glass vigorously and take a teaspoon of the mixture once every ten minutes.

I did that and by the time I was seen by the doctor in the hospital, my headache had vanished. In fact, he was quite annoyed that I had wasted his time, and I do not blame him. He had not seen me one hour previously, and he had not had the good fortune to discover homeopathy. How was he to know that a minor stroke of magic had just taken place?

**I often tell patients to plus remedies when the potency they were using for an acute that runs out of steam**. I find, by plussing remedies in the way I was first instructed, the remedy often works again, although sometimes the next potency up the scale is required to complete the cure.

Several homeopaths I interviewed for the second part of this book have suggested that dissolving a remedy in water without succession makes a remedy gentler and less aggravating.

# POTENCY AND REMEDY

The meeting of minds is very important in homeopathic education. It is sometimes possible to weave someone else's discoveries with one's own and grow richer. This diffusion has happened to me after each interview. Anthony Bickley was my very first interviewee on the subject of potency and dosage.

When I first contacted him, I remember he asked me who else I had approached. I said that I had contacted Rajan Sankaran, but sadly he had declined the offer of speaking to me. Anthony then said 'I'm sure my opinions are nothing like Sankaran's!'

Well, Anthony, maybe not. But your experience of potency certainly complements an idea of Sankaran's about the sycotic miasm, and an idea of mine that has already been expressed.

Let me explain:

Anthony is not alone in thinking that the remedy you use dictates the potency. I have heard through the grapevine (from one of his students) that a particular lecturer, for example, always gives *Opium* in a low potency. Presumably because an *Opium* patient is expected to exhibit low energy. When one is fixed in this way, it does limit the options when choosing a potency, but I can certainly see where this idea comes from.

Anthony goes further with this idea. He takes into account the nature of the remedy and the miasm when choosing a potency. As described in his interview, he gives patients who need remedies of the sycotic miasm a lower dose. Here the miasm helps dictate the choice of potency.

Rajan Sankaran speaks of the sycotic miasm as having something to hide. If, therefore, patients have something to hide, practitioners are not always able to discover what they are hiding. We often feel we are being kept in the dark about something, and that our remedy choice is inaccurate. This is a very good reason for choosing a lower potency.

With Rajan's influence, this would also make me seek a sycotic remedy. Now, we are coming round in circles, but do you see what I mean? Anthony and I are coming from very different places, but in essence, it appears we are both doing the same thing!

Interestingly, Anthony Bickley and Rajan Sankaran suggest that as a patient gets healthier, the potency is reduced.

I do not wish to say any more on this subject. I would rather the reader find the threads that link the theories and discoveries together. It is my opinion that Anthony Bickley has something important to teach us that can make us better homeopaths. My experience has not led me to think of the nature of the remedy and miasm when choosing a potency, but I will now. I also think that our pooled experiences as homeopaths are far greater than our individual findings, and this is just one example of it all coming together.

# POTENCY AND SUPPRESSION

Suppression is just another way of saying hidden or controlled. Collins English Dictionary's (Millennium Edition) definition of 'to suppress' is:
a)  To put an end to; prohibit
b)  To hold in check; restrain
c)  To resist consciously
d)  To exercise control by preventing the expression of

**It makes sense to me to use lower potencies in suppressed cases**, for reasons already discussed in the previous chapter. Suppressed cases need you to go gently because you are never quite sure what you are going to bring out.  Prescribing for such cases, one is almost certainly going to provoke some sort of aggravation at some point. If something has been suppressed, whether it is a symptom like eczema from cortisone cream or an emotional experience that someone does not want to face, it is going to have to come out in order for that person to move on. In my view it is important that both the practitioner and the patient anticipate this.  But just how fast and furiously this happens, depends on  the practitioner, partly on how attached the patient is to his suppression, and partly on the patient/practitioner relationship.

However, the patients' experience of homeopathy in these cases does not have to be all doom and gloom.  As energy is transferred to their system via the most appropriate remedy at the time, there is a strengthening of the vital force happening too.  In my experience, many things can generally improve when patients with suppressed conditions receive less deep remedies. In the beginning it can seem that even the main complaint is getting better. Then at some point - and it could be at the beginning, or it could be after a long while the focus seems to grow more and more on the actual problem, heightening it until the simillimum becomes obvious and begs to be found.

**I have found that low potencies at the outset will be the gentlest approach,** the patient will feel the benefit of them and choose to continue with homeopathy.  **Low and often usually works best, especially for people who are on medication, except for those with sensitive constitutions.**  Then as the patient becomes more energised from his remedies, his problem will become clearer, he will be less sick and the information for finding the simillimum will become more accessible. If the simillimum, or a close enough remedy, is not given at the most acute stage, then his suffering will continue.  If a close enough replica to his problem is not found at this stage, the patient has more energy to express himself but his main complaint is highlighted and feels worse. I have found that if the simillimum or a very close remedy is administered in such circumstances, a low dose can sometimes do a wonderful job, while a high dose has the power to perform a miraculous result.

# POTENCY AND TROUBLESHOOTING

I want to speak a bit more about potency in situations when remedies throw up an intensity of symptoms that appear like an acute, where the homeopath feels he must act quickly. It tends to happen when the patient reacts intensely to the first remedy he receives, or when energy has been thrown into the system by a close remedy or a series of close remedies. In the second instance the patient appears at first to be healing but keeps relapsing, until at one time he lapses quite dramatically (see Case 12).

## CASE TWELVE
*Female*
*12 years*

**18.01.02**

*Presenting: emotional problems*

*Finds it hard to fall asleep. Goes to bed at 9pm and doesn't fall asleep till 11.30pm and sometimes later. Is tired in the morning.*

*Is a worrier (tears), wants to be cuddled by mum, panics if mum is not there. If mum goes round the corner she panics. (These are mum's observations, patient herself says she doesn't panic, she just likes being with mum all the time.) Doesn't like to go to friends' houses to sleep. Prefers to sleep at home.*

*Has just started a new school. Has had to make all new friends. There's been a few tears at school. Feels sick in the car on the way in.*

*To live with, she's talkative and very kind. Every other word is 'I love you mummy'. Mum feels she is always attention seeking. She talks to mum from another room, for example, just to check mum is still in there. As a baby, was needy for only mum. Is very sensitive. Procrastinates if asked to do something.*

*Her room has to be tidy. She likes to be organised with school homework and things. Is very good with her homework. It's the first thing she does when she comes home. She likes to please people.*

*Fears: spiders, being alone (says she can fall asleep better if someone is in the room with her).*

*There's often tears at bed-time because she's worried about the next day. She feels like a lost soul at school, even though her two brothers are there. She feels she doesn't know anybody very well yet. She is not worried about the work.*

*Dreams: running across a rainbow.*
*Her dog having puppies.*
*Someone in the house chasing her which she says wasn't scary.*

*Often gets headaches on arriving home from school.*

### Repertorisation:

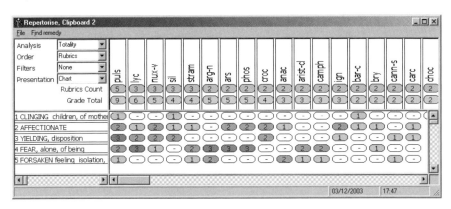

**Prescription**: *Pulsatilla 1M daily for 3 days (standard dosage for me at the time of prescribing), because I thought the remedy was obvious enough.*

### 19.02.02

*Is now going to bed at between 9.30 and 10pm, without tears falls asleep more or less straight away. Is not tired in the mornings.*

*Dreams: of Gareth in Pop Idol, but can't remember much about it.*

*Her clinginess has been better. Is worrying though. Has to organise everything. Everything has to be just so. Does everything in advance, like getting her clothes out before going to bed. Needs it all organised.*

*Just after had the remedy, started to tell mum everything. If something is on her mind gets very tearful. Becomes all consumed with guilt. She verbally repeats herself, or if she moves a chair then she must move it again. If she says something, she is worried about saying the wrong thing. Is worried about hurting people. Would be upset that they wouldn't like her. Doesn't like anyone to be upset or cross with her. If they are she will apologise profusely and be over the top with it.*

*Mum says she doesn't want to sleep at someone else's house, nor does she want a friend to come and sleep over at her house.*

*She hasn't had many headaches, only one or two since we last met.*

**Comment:** *some improvement, therefore no prescription at present. However, something else is emerging since the remedy that is not Pulsatilla.*

### 25.03.02

*Doing really well at school now and sleeping better. Is a constant chatterbox and mumbles to herself. A bit more clingy. Asks mum if she'd like a cup of tea many times, even after mum has consistently said no. Can't make a decision for herself. No headaches. Is not so tearful.*

### Repertorisation:

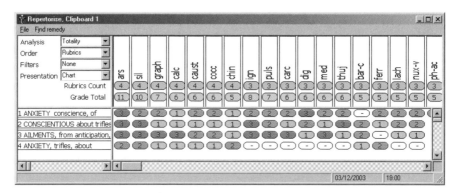

**Comment:** *anxious, tearful, must tell all her problems to mum, fastidious, irresolute: this made me think of Graphites. Although*

*everything was seemingly pointing to this remedy, it did not feel quite right, however I had nothing better to give her at the time.*

**Prescription**: *Graphites 200c daily for three days. Dosage was standard, potency was chosen because I originally thought of an 1M as all the mentals/emotionals were there, but then I gave a lower potency because of my gut feeling that it was not quite right.*

**22.04.02**

*Unhappy. Complains of too much homework and doesn't always want to do it, and if she doesn't do it, will only have more the next day. Is worried about getting it all done. Hasn't got the time to do everything at night.*

*Has become tearful at school. Has to do things twice and that leaves her behind at school.*

*If someone questions her, even if she's in the right, still feels guilty and wrong. If she upsets someone they might not like her and that wouldn't be very nice.*

*It would be nice not to worry about anything. Would worry if she did something that she was not supposed to do. Worries and feels guilty about different things that she can't tell me. Doesn't forgive herself. Tries to ignore these things and not think about them.*

*Observation: she's wringing her hands and playing with her fingers.*

*Mum's observations: doesn't like anyone to come between mum and herself. If mum goes out, she will ask how long mum will be. Often says 'stop looking at me', and asks mum questions that she already knows the answer to.*

*Mum encouraged her to tell me what she felt guilty about. She cheated in an exam, and she pretended her teddy bears were boyfriends.*

*She says that there are other things she's done that she shouldn't have, and she feels guilty and worried about them too. 'I just want to be normal.'*

**Repertorisation:**

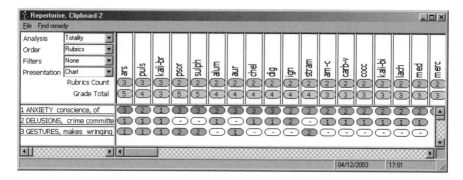

**Prescription**: Kali bromatum 1M daily for 3 days.

**Comment**: Secretiveness, guilt and morality. Kali Bromatum. It felt like I'd at last got to the centre of the case, and I went higher in potency.

### 18.06.02

Feeling a lot happier. Less clingy to mum and doing well at school. Still tells mum 'I love you' a lot, and asks 'Are you sure you love me?'

Still has to do things twice, though homework is not such a problem. Hasn't had such strong feelings around guilt. Still would rather be with family than friends. Doesn't want to sleep over with friends. Gets homesick. Misses mum. Likes being at home. Always a panic 'What time will you pick me up?' or 'You will be there won't you?'

When she was small, would cling to mum's leg and no-one could come between her and mum. Doesn't like to be away from home because doesn't feel secure. Is not good at making decisions either. Is defensive, bashful and shy.

## Repertorisation:

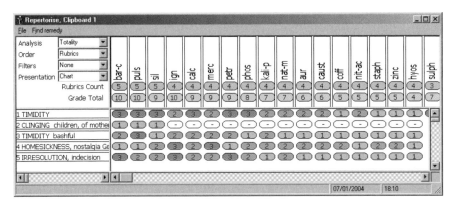

**Comment**: Baryta carb? On reflection I can see that I was losing the thread of the case. At the time I must have felt fairly sure of the prescription as patient was expressing less guilt and more lack of self confindence.

**Prescription**: Baryta carb 200c daily for 3 days.


### 02.08.02

Been more sociable. More adventurous. Not panicking when mum goes out.


**Comment:** things seemed to be moving in the right direction. Her confidence has picked up. No mention of the guilt and ritualistic behaviour. I therefore decided to wait.


### 02.09.02

She has gone back to how she was.

Had a panic attack when stayed with grandma. Was thumping her chest and saying that her heart was hurting.

Is waking mum up at night and wanting to sleep on the floor by mum's bed. Been quite lethargic and apathetic. Is checking things again. Everything must be repeated, done twice.

Is lacking in confidence, insecure and hanging off mum's leg. Is constantly chattering. Keeps saying pardon because wants mum to say things twice. Says the same things in ten different ways. Feels as if has to do it. Talks a lot and waffles. If doesn't repeat things believes she'll have bad luck. Feels compelled to tell mum everything and ask everything.

**Comment**: I was confused. I felt I was getting the result of a problem but not going behind it, despite my probing. This compulsion was not easy for mum or patient to stand. I felt I had to do something, so I gave Thuja. The main essence of Thuja being to hide one's true and therefore flawed nature and cover it up with behaviour that characterises what they think they should be. One of the expressions of this coping structure going wrong can be ritualistic behaviour. I also have known a prescription of Thuja to give the patient the ability to express themselves more openly. Fairly confident that I was doing the right thing at that moment, I opted for the 200c potency.

**Prescription:** Thuja 200c daily for 3 days.

### 10.01.03

Hasn't been to see me for the last three months because was 100% better. Now, since last week, has gone full circle.

Everything has been about death. Ghosts might haunt me. If I think something it might happen. Has become superstitious. A little boy died near where they live, and patient asks mum if he'll go to heaven or hell. Is very anxious. 'If I think it, it will come true. It's all down to me. I must lie with my feet and hands together, if I move them, then it might happen.' Sometimes when spells something must spell it backwards for things to be alright.

Gets panic stricken. Says to mum 'You decide' and wants mum to make it alright.

If has bad thoughts about the baby (mum's pregnant), she thinks they will come true. Feels her thoughts are responsible for things happening.

Is not eating much.

Dreamt she had been raped and felt disgusted at having such a thought.

I asked her what type of person would have these thoughts and she replied, 'a witch'.

**Comment**: Thuja worked in an interesting way, firstly by ameliorating the situation, and then making the picture more obvious and to the point. I felt at this juncture, I ought to know the remedy, but did not, and yet here was the opportunity I was waiting for. In desperation, I tried Kola (dreams of witches[6] and has feelings of self- disgust[7]), Cyclamen (for the guilt aspect) and Rhus Tox (Superstitiousness), waiting only days between each prescription. I was clutching at straws and knew it. In the meantime things got so bad, my patient couldn't stand it anymore. The guilt and the compulsive behaviour reached a fever pitch and mum took her to the doctor and received a prescription for Seroxat. When I actually found the simillimum, by exploring the repertory, first by doing a search in 'Isis' for the word 'witch', then 'magic', and finally going through every remedy in the rubric 'superstitious'. Mancinella was confirmed to me in an article in Links magazine[8] that is loaded onto my computer, the cured cases in that article mirrored this case perfectly and if she had not been on allopathic medication, I would have given a very high dose, instead I gave an LM specifically because she was on medication.

**Prescription**: Mancinella LM1

**Comment:** patient has been doing very well since January. At first she had the thoughts, but felt she did not have to act on them. This was the effect of Seroxat, I think. Then as the remedy took hold, the thoughts gradually reduced. I am hoping she will reduce her allopathic medication soon.

The homeopath must find a suitable remedy quickly when there is an intensity of symptoms and often takes the presenting symptoms as they stand. If the homeopath prescribes well, he or she is likely, at this point, to find a deeply curative remedy for the patient's pathology.

In these instances, I usually prescribe as if the patient has a sort of semi-acute. If the state is very intense and the characteristic symptoms very strong, I will go high, and have been known to do wonders with a 50M daily for three days. Very often I will give a 200c daily, for up to five days, when the symptoms are less vivid, going up in potency later if need be. I tend to keep in touch with the patient during this period, to

---

[6] *The Complete Repertory*

[7] *An Insight into Plants* by Rajan Sankaran

[8] *Links* 1/93 page 9-12 article titled 'Children's remedies' by Vassilis Ghegas

ensure that we are turning things around. **The benchmark for potency and dosage is the intensity and vivacity and vividness of the situation. If the patient choosing to go on allopathic medication has already suppressed the symptoms, I will generally go lower, use an LM,** and review in a month.

# STRANGE DISCOVERIES WITH POTENCY

It takes time to build up one's confidence as a homeopath, at least it did for me. During my first five years in practice, I would assume that if the remedy did not work, then it was the wrong remedy. Then along came a case to challenge that hypothesis:

## CASE THIRTEEN
*Female*
*5 months old*

### 09.06.98

*Presenting complaint: Cough.*

*Started coughing ten weeks previously, after vaccination. Barking cough and she makes a very strange noise after coughing. Had been coughing and bringing up every feed. OK between feeds except for sleepiness. Goes red in the face with cough. Rattling of mucus in throat and vomiting mucus.*

*Usually very happy and easy baby.*

**Prescription:** DPT 30c sd

**Comment:** *I gave this prescription based on aetiology only. I do not usually prescribe like this, but wanted to see if it would work for us in this instance.*

### 12.06.98

*No change*

**Prescription**: Thuja 200c sd

**Comment:** *once again I was giving this remedy based on aetiology, and the rubric 'Cough after Vaccination', in which Thuja is the only remedy to appear. Growing more sure of my prescription, I decided to up the potency.*

**16.06.98**

*Cough improved slightly, followed by a worsening by 18.06.98.*

*Other remedies tried unsuccessfully were Antimonium tartaricum 30c (rattling respiration) Phosphorous 30c (cough, plus usually a very happy and easy baby), Tuberculinum 30c (the remedy for respiratory complaints).*

**16.12.98**

*I received a letter from the patient's mum to say that the baby had been poorly on and off since we'd spoken last and had been admitted twice into Barnet General Hospital with breathing difficulties and her 'spectacular' cough.*

**15.03.99**

*Mum phoned me again. The cough still was no better and is there anything else I can think of to help. This time I took the original symptoms and repertorised them. Was the sound she make after coughing a whoop?*

**Repertorisation:**

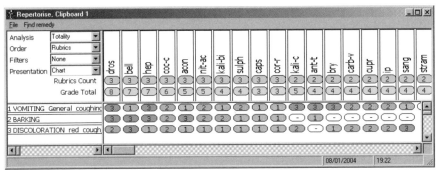

**Prescription:** *gave Drosera 200c. This helped slightly, then mum plussed the remedy, but it no longer helped.*

**20.04.99**

*Gave Thuja LM1 daily and this proved to be curative.*

*This patient's cough returned one year later and Drosera 1M seemed to clear it up a second time, and a third time one year after that.*

**What I had learned from this case was that not only does finding the correct remedy count, but potency and dosage are important too.** Perhaps if I would have stuck with *Thuja* 200c in the beginning and repeated it, or perhaps if I had gone from *Drosera* 200c to 1M in the first instance, then things might have improved faster. I will never know.

Interestingly, both those two very different remedies had an impact; *Thuja* from an aetiological point of view was indicated and Drosera, because it fitted the cough. I wonder if *Thuja* 200c was too high in potency and that is why things worsened after an initial amelioration? If this is so, it would fit in with my idea that lower potencies are better if the match is only partial, and *Drosera*, being a better picture of what she was expressing, actually needed a higher potency to make it work well.

I was learning. Learning to trust myself. Learning to question every response or lack of it to a prescription. 'What happened there?' was the question I frequently asked myself. 'Why did that remedy not work in that potency?' 'Am I sure I want to change the remedy?' 'What about the potency?' Mostly I want to change the remedy, but changing the potency is on the list of options now, and it always, if it is appropriate, proves curative.

# CASE FOURTEEN
*Male*
*6 years*

*I had a call from the mother of one of my patients, a child. Her son had a high temperature and was exuding heat. She had tried Belladonna and it had not helped. I questioned her further to see if there were any more symptoms. All the symptoms that he was exhibiting were Belladonna symptoms: fever, exuding heat, thirstless, cold extremities etc., I asked about potency, and she revealed she had given him Belladonna 200c.*

**Comment:** *in the absence of mental and emotional symptoms, I decided that it fitted my 'superficial' category (SEE CHAPTER ON SUPERFICIALITY page 28). I told the mum to try Belladonna 30c hourly for three to four hours and phone me. When I spoke to her next, the temperature had come down nicely, and by the following day my patient was well enough to go back to school.*

The above experience of using a lower potency to get a remedy to work in an acute where the symptoms all point to a remedy but the picture is 'superficial', has been repeated many times. It often happens when a mum has prescribed on the picture first and called me when the remedy has not worked. So far, bringing down the potency in these circumstances has never failed me.

I have had similar experiences when I have prescribed the wrong potency in chronic cases.

# CASE FIFTEEN
*Female*
*10 years old*

**03.09.02**

*(I had previously treated this patient for a chronic cough and used the remedy* Calcarea carbonica *successfully, but as in other cases already depicted in this book, something else was emerging. The early part of the case has nothing to demonstrate by way of potency, so I'm starting it from the fourth time I'd seen her).*

Hasn't been getting to sleep since her holiday. Was jet lagged when she came home. Woke up a few days after her holiday with a nightmare. Was frightened about the two girls who had recently gone missing (on the news). The nightmare was about this, and this news story has been on her mind a lot. She worries and she panics.

*'I can't get to sleep. I'm congested and I'm hot.'*

Sometimes she stands on the stairs and moans like a three year old. Once mum sits on her bed for four or five minutes, she goes to sleep. Needs the comfort of mum being there. Worries if mum goes out in the evening that she's not going to come home.

Everything has got to be in the right place before she goes to sleep. Everything must be put away or if she can't find a place for it, it has to be taken out of the room. Generally, there's a lot of tidying before she goes to sleep and she is a bit of a hoarder.

Mum says she wants everyone to think that she is perfect. Doesn't like her bad side to be revealed. Gets very disappointed if someone sees her other side. Everything may be tidy on the surface, but her drawers and cupboards are a mess.

## Repertorisation:

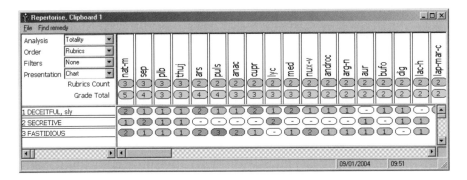

**Assessment**: this originally seemed to me like an Arsenicum album state, but based on what mum said in the last paragraph, I gave Thuja. I used the 1M potency because I felt sure of the prescription at the time, although there were obvious elements of Arsenicum album to be observed, in other cases I have often pondered whether to give Thuja or Arsenicum album. The deciding factor, in this instance was, that she is tidy only on the surface. I would like to refer the reader to the chapters on Thuja in Vermeulen's Synoptic Materia Medica, Volume one, and Sankaran's The Soul of Remedies.

**Prescription:** Thuja 1M sd


### 04.11.02

Has had two tummy aches and a couple of headaches. Has had to take rescue remedy occasionally. Has to phone mum if she goes out on a Saturday night, and always says that something is wrong. Afterwards apologises for not allowing mum to enjoy herself. Always asks, 'How long will you be out and what time are you coming home?'

Everything in her room has to be just so. If something is out of place must put it right. She bosses her little brother around and has been a lot more argumentative recently. Her verruca was gone.

Question: why does she feel the need to phone mum?

Answer: because she misses her and gets very worried and panicky. Used to think that someone will bang through the door.

### Repertorisation:

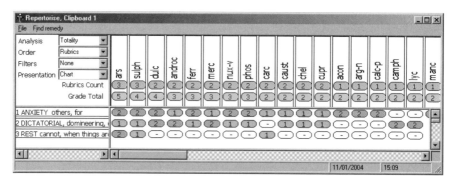

**Prescription:** Arsenicum album 1M daily for 3 days

**Comment:** Remedy given because case is starting to look more like Arsenicum, and therefore a high potency is given.

### 17.12.02

Headaches went and came back. Tummy aches have gone.
It's fine for mum to go out during the week, but not on weekends. Told the babysitter, 'If I can make myself upset then mum won't go out'.

'I don't like it when she goes out. It feels weird when she's not there and she doesn't put me to bed. When she's not around it's different. During the week I know where she's going. Saturday night, I don't know anything. I like knowing where she goes. I normally see her during the week and she gives me a kiss goodnight. On Saturday night, I don't see her. During the week, I can see her when she gets back. If I wake up I like to see her there. If mum is not in the house I get panicky. I can't get to sleep and I get worried. I don't get panicky if mum's there. It has to be either mum or dad at home'.

Question: What are you panicking about?

Answer: I have everything going through my mind: what time will they come home; that something might happen in the car; or they might not get back. They may break down and not come home, and then I wouldn't see them.

Question : Then what would happen?

*Answer: If I don't get to see them, I'll get upset. I can't say 'Hello, did you have a nice evening', and they can't put me into bed. I'd get nervous and worried if they got home very late. The next morning I'll be tired because I couldn't get to sleep. Even if I think of something exciting, I still can't get to sleep.*

*Sometimes I phone her and can't get a connection. I worry that they can get hurt. I worry they might not be all right. I worry that they are not safe and I must stay up to make sure they get home safely. Sometimes I like them to keep me safe.*

*Her mum says: she feels dread when she goes out. Hates having to report home every five minutes. Mum feels the whole thing is a control issue. Her daughter doesn't think she should go out, and is becoming aggressive and mouthy. She answers back. If she doesn't like what mum's saying, she puts her hands up to stop her speaking. If mum says something, she asks mum to be quiet because mum is embarrassing her. Everything must be in its right place to keep her happy. She likes to go to bed in mum's bed because she feels more secure there. She's always kissing mum and telling her how much she loves her. She is mothering her brother as well!*

**Comment**: *Arsenicum, Arsenicum, Arsenicum, and yet, it didn't do anything.*

**Prescription:** *I gave Arsenicum album 10M daily for 3 days.*

### 14.01.03

*No head aches. No tummy aches.*

*Been absolutely fine when mum goes out. Is feeling better about things. Still says a few things and phones mum when she's out to find out when she will return. Hasn't panicked or suggested mum doesn't go out or return home. Still must have everything in the right place. Is aggressive at times but on the whole more loving. Mum reports a massive improvement.*

*The case continues.*

# CASE SIXTEEN

*Female*
*9 years*

*(Once again, I'm going to begin this case in the middle, as this is a child I have seen on and off for a while and previous case taking is irrelevant when it comes down to demonstrating the potency.)*

### 13.07.01

*Having headaches. Feels dizzy and it hurts. Has to rest her head on her legs or put her head on the desk.*

*Has dreams about the babysitter. People trying to shoot people in the bank. The dreams are scary.*

*The headaches make her feel sick.*

*Often thinks there is someone in the house at night. Has to check the windows ten times to see they are not open. Worries if the shower door is not closed perfectly. Has to check everything to see it is as it should be.*

*Wants everyone to be safe. Gets worried if mum and dad talk about people dying.*

### Repertorisation:

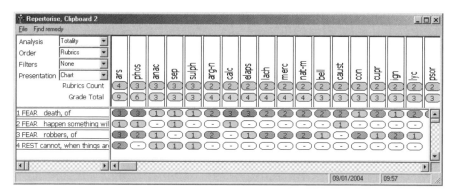

**Prescription**: Arsenicum album 1M daily for three days.

**Comment:** *I was sure of the prescription and therefore gave a high potency. One a day for three days was standard for me at the time.*

## 17.12.01

*Headaches are better.*

*Still checking the windows and looking under the bed and in the cupboards. Wakes two to three times a night then goes back to sleep. Scared at night.*

*Keeps thinking a lady from an advert is behind her. Wouldn't like to wait for mum in the car and worries about being kidnapped.*

*Thinks someone's hand will come out if doesn't check the cupboards and drawers.*

*Worries about burglars and robbers.*

*Has dreams of being killed and being taken away in her sleep and no-one could find her. Whenever dad is away on business, is frightened because mum is not a man. Likes her room tidy but doesn't care about the rest of the house. It bothers her at night if things are not in the right place, but doesn't care during the day.*

**Comment:** *her headaches disappeared after the Arsenicum album 1M, but her fears seemed to be heightened, so on the 14.08.01, I gave Arsenicum album 10M. Nothing happened. I saw hints of the sycotic miasm in the case when she said that she thinks someone is following her (keeps thinking a lady from an advert is behind her). On 19.0./01 I gave Thuja 1M. Nothing happened. I thought I would give Arsenicum album one more try. I was starting to wonder if she would benefit from repeated doses. Not wishing to give a high potency often, I decided to try an LM.*

**Prescription:** Arsenicum album LM1

## 05.02.02

*Still checking windows, but not checking everything. Not frantically checking things like she was before. Has had no bad dreams.*

**Prescription**: *Arsenicum LM2*


**24.04.02**

*She is not checking anything anymore and her fears seems to have all abated.*

*She says: I never check things or wake up in the night anymore. That's babyish.*


**Comment:** *why the higher potencies did not work in this instance might have been because I was prescribing 'superficially', and therefore only seeing part of a picture. Indeed, whenever I saw this patient, I always had her two other siblings to find remedies for, and there never seemed to be enough concentrated time for her. However, the LM worked well.*


Alize Timmerman spoke at the Society Conference a couple of years ago and briefly told us of her discovery. She spoke of a *Natrum mur - iaticum* patient, and how she was so certain that the patient needed *Natrum muriaticum*, but the remedy did not work in any potency that she tried. She ended up making up the remedy in a different way and finally it worked. (SEE INTERVIEW WITH ALIZE TIMMERMAN page 215)

# STRANGE DISCOVERIES WITH AGGRAVATIONS

It was about five years ago that someone suggested using a 6c to bring down an aggravation. Nowadays, **if I have given a high or fairly high centesimal potency and the patient has more intense symptoms (but the same symptoms), I think of giving a single dose of that remedy in a 6c, and the aggravation usually lessens pretty quickly.**

Here are two examples of this:

## CASE SEVENTEEN
*Male*
*7 years old*

### 28.11.00

*Presenting: asthma since four years.*

*Hugely fluctuating mood swings. Very impatient. Very highly strung. Hot and cold moods. His motor skills are not great.*

*When he gets a cold it leads to asthma. Is coughing at the moment.*

*Sleeps well, mum says. He says, 'How do you know, you don't even know how I sleep.' Gets very sweaty at night and likes mum or dad to read to him before sleep. It takes about two hours for him to fall asleep. He's a restless sleeper and is tired on waking.*

*Dreams: used to have terrifying nightmares.*

*He craves sweets.*

*Fears: Scary movies. Gory things. Hides under the covers, but doesn't need the light on. He talks a lot about murder. Asks things like, where do gladiators get stabbed? Last year talked about hurricanes and floods. He says, 'My dad tells me some quite bad things'. Mum and dad did bad things. They let me see (the film) The Mummy.*

*Observation: he doesn't look at me when he speaks to me, and he is drawing a vivid picture of a torture chamber with someone being tortured.*

*He says he worries about being an angel because he wouldn't like to be an angel.*

*Mum says he has a strong personality. Draining at times. Very challenging. When he makes up his mind, that's it. If mum wants him to do something, there are tears, he throws things and kicks things, swears and bites. At times the whole family has to walk on eggshells.*

*His triggers are: His brother. If his brother has something that he hasn't. It can be attention seeking. Or if another child touches his toy.*

*He is a hoarder: 'He squirrels things away'.*

*At school he is making good progress, but his attention span is an on-going problem, and he is restless in his chair.*

*He lacks confidence. If he is not sure how to spell a word, will say that he can't do it. He is afraid to get things wrong. Lots of one-upmanship. With his work, he gets very frustrated and says 'I'm the stupidest kid in the world'.*

*He never forgets a name or a face. He's very competitive with his brother for dad's attention.*

*He was an easy baby. He slept through the night at seven weeks old. He was really fine until his brother came along.*

*He often says 'Mummy doesn't like me/love me and she thinks I'm the stupidest kid in the world'.*

*He's very affectionate with his dad. When he does something, the details he goes into are amazing.*

*He says, 'I wish I was a bat. It's the bat's lucky day. He killed all the people and ate the blood'.*

*He has a low sensory threshold. Gets angry if there are wrinkles in his socks, if the seams are not straight, and he only likes to wear particular shirts. He fears loud noises and smells everything.*

*He doesn't like change. He likes to know where he is going. He likes predictability, and doesn't like alterations in his plans. He can feel shy with other kids. He dribbles at night. Sometimes he lies on the floor and wriggles around. He has a perpetually stuffy nose.*

*He's cautious. Knows how to avoid dangerous situations. He's agile and confident in the playground. Not reckless but calculated. He is very trustworthy when it comes to safety.*

*He would like to change his brother. 'I want to change him to dead.'*

**Comment:** *at first, I gave him Lachesis, but I wasn't sure about it and therefore wanted to prescribe low, also something about his strength of character made me choose an LM; I thought he might fight the influence of the remedy and would therefore benefit from repeated doses. I thought if the remedy is not quite right a repeated low dose just might make an impression. My reasons for giving Lachesis were 1. His thoughts of evil and fear of evil. 2. His love of power. 3. Horrible things affect him profoundly. 4. There is an aetiology of his brother's birth and the desire for his brother to be dead 5. The night sweats and the wriggling on the floor (like a snake).*

**Repertorisation:**

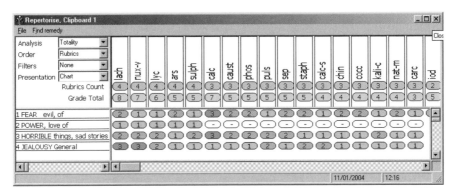

**Prescription:** Lachesis LM1

### 18.12.00

*Has a tight wheezy cough, especially at night. Hasn't been ill at all. Has had to use his inhaler once.*

*He's been very oppositional. Very contrary. Everything is an argument. He wants to make all the decisions and control everything. He likes to* do controversial drawings (like the torture chamber) and say things to get a reaction.

He can scream for no reason and grunt...

**Comment:** I don't think the Lachesis has done very much, if anything at all. I'm not happy with keeping him on the same remedy. There are things about the case which are not really characteristic of Lachesis, like his hypersensitivity to noise, smell, stimulus, and his fear of failure.

**Prescription:** Feeling pretty sure of my remedy this time, I gave Nux vomica 1M daily for three days.

### 26.01.01

Eczema and coughing 75% improved.

Has a bit of a dry tickly cough in the evenings, but it never progresses beyond that. His nose is not so stuffy. His contrariness is better. He is much more agreeable, and seems more content.

He still does things for shock value, but his outbursts of swearing are fewer and further between. He is less brooding and brighter. He still likes to be in charge and is still hot at night, but much better about going to sleep. He is tired, but more agreeable on waking...

**Comment:** of course I should have waited, but in a moment of madness I gave him more remedy and upped the potency. What was I thinking?

**Prescription:** Nux vomica 10M daily for three days

**Comment:** very soon after that I got a phone call from mum that his asthma had 'kicked in really badly'. I immediately gave Nux vomica 6c in a single dose and that seemed to get us back on the right track within a very short space of time. By the 27.03.01 he reached a space where he was not coughing at all and his emotional/behavioural self was continuing to improve. The family emigrated and I have not heard from them since.

Finally, and most controversially, I have recently had an experience whereby when I went down in potency the patient aggravated. The case is as follows:


## CASE EIGHTEEN

*Female*
*35 years old*

*(I had been treating this patient on and off for a couple of years. Remedies helped in acute situations and with other problems, but in the grand scheme of things nothing moved her on dynamically and she remained somewhat of an enigma to me remedy-wise, until the consultation that took place in May 2002.)*


**20.05.02**

*Has lost control (patient in tears).*
*Very high anxiety all the time.*
*Has lost one and a half stone and her hair is falling out.*
*Permanently thinks the kids are ill.*
*Goes into a complete panic over little things they suffer from.*
*'I can't go on like this. I'm absolutely drained. I've been fighting it so long, I've no strength left anymore.'*

*When at work can turn off. 'I swing the other way. I get excited about going to work. It's like before going on holiday.'*

*Her husband is picky and a hard person. When she used to be relaxed, he'd get picky. So now, she never relaxes. Feels tense and rigid, so when the girls are ill she won't feel as if she's been hit. 'Because it's a real hit like a punch in the stomach.' Has to keep one step ahead the whole time...*


**Comment:** *she'd only been speaking for about ten minutes, but I was already certain about the remedy she needed. I therefore decided a high potency was called for. The dosage of daily for three days was standard for me at the time.*

In terms of my decision for giving the remedy, once again I would like to refer the reader to Rajan Sankaran's *Soul of Remedies*[9], where he says of Rhus Tox that this remedy can 'face some kind of danger of attack from members of his own family...he always has to be on his guard...and has a constant anxiety 'as if something is going to happen'.

**Prescription:** Rhus tox 10M daily for three days

## 17.06.02

*Is so much better. 'Within three days I felt normal. After the second day the energy was rushing through my body and everything lifted. Everything: It's amazing.'*

*'Last week I felt slightly anxious again. I still have a slightly short fuse if something doesn't go my way. I've put on weight and am eating again. I'm like a different person since I took the remedy.'*

**Comment:** *It was a wonderful response, but because she had started to feel slightly anxious again, I repeated the remedy.*

**Prescription:** *Rhus Tox 10M single dose.*

**Comment:** *I also had cause to repeat the remedy once more on the 9.09.2002.*

## 16.10.02

*'For the last couple of weeks, I've felt panicky in the mornings. I am feeling a bit sick again like I used to. I've had a headache and I haven't had one for months and months. It's the same feeling, I think the kids are ill when they are not...'*

**Comment:** *I knew that I had to repeat the remedy, but was concerned that whereas the penultimate dose lasted around three months, this last dose only held for approximately one month. Under normal circumstances, I would have increased the potency at this point, but had read somewhere that the correct thing to do is decrease the*

---

[9] *The Soul of Remedies* by Rajan Sankaran, page 173

*potency as the patient's health improved, and I was in an experimental mood.*

**Prescription:** Rhus Tox 1M

## Phone call 21.10.02

*Has a burning mouth. Lips sore, especially when she licks them. Lips are puffy too. She now has a rash all over her neck and feels generally lousy.*

## Phone call 24.10.02

*No improvement.*

**Prescription:** Rhus Tox 6c sd

## Phone call 28.10.02

*Things have started to improve.*

## Phone call 30.10.02

*Feeling panicky. Fears the children being ill. Was dizzy yesterday. Skin is peeling and very sore. Has a bitter taste in her mouth, and all food tastes bitter.*

**Prescription:** Aconite 30c sd

**Comment:** *after the Aconite, things steadily improved, but this case has certainly taught me a few lessons. Firstly, I have never had this kind of problem with ascending the potency as the patient's health improves, so descending the potency in this way is not something I wish to try again. Secondly, lower potencies are not necessarily gentler potencies. In fact, as far as I am concerned, the only gentle potency is an appropriate potency. And thirdly, interestingly enough, did you notice that the 6c potency did seem to work to turn the aggravation around, even though it would have been less troublesome, I believe, to* *have given a higher potency in the first place? Perhaps the most aggravating potencies therefore, are the ones immediately above and below the appropriate potency. In other words a bit too high or a bit too low is when we stimulate too aggressively.*

On reading Rajan Sankaran's new book *An Insight into Plants*, I noticed a case where a good general response occurred after the remedy *Chocolate* 200c was administered, but the patient's migraine headaches increased. The headaches only went away after a dose of *Chocolate* 1M.[10]

Another case in the same book aggravated terribly after a lower potency, but did not seem to when higher potencies were subsequently given.[11]

I am sure there are many more examples to be found that demonstrate high is not necessarily aggressive, but the opposite. Nevertheless, all of the above three cases suggest that **a lower potency can cause havoc if it is not the right potency, whereas an ideal higher potency can be a gentler cure**. Mike Bridger seems to agree with this; see his interview in part two of this book (page 159).

---

[10] *An Insight into Plants* by Rajan Sankaran, pages 636-640
[11] *Ibid*, pages559-566

# READING AGGRAVATIONS

Let us be specific now. What exactly is an aggravation? I would say that an aggravation is where energy has been put into the system and caused havoc, and sometimes that havoc goes on to cure.

So, how can we tell if it will or not?

I think the answer depends on how the aggravation presents itself. In my experience if the vital force is met by a similar disease agent but too high in potency, then one of two things can happen. Either the patient experiences a symptom as if he/she has been on a detox diet and the body is throwing out waste, e.g. a skin rash, headache, boil, diarrhoea. In fact, any symptom where the person is clearly getting rid of something. Or, there is an intensification of the symptoms he is already experiencing. With either of these, if I have originally given a centesimal potency, I will give a lower potency, as I was taught, a 6c.

In this circumstance, it is as if the excess of energy in the remedy illuminates the picture greatly for a while before finally dimming the subjective symptoms of the patient. A lower potency can act as a high-speed dimmer in these situations.

However, I do expect these types of aggravations to start improving pretty quickly, especially if the intensity is difficult for the patient to bear. If they do not, I normally re-take the case, hoping to find a more similar remedy to that which the vital force is currently expressing. This is in keeping with what Hahnemann advocated in the *Organon*. aphorisms 167 & 170. The potency for the new remedy will generally be higher too, as the patient throws up this semi-acute, his vital force is re-energised and he has the newborn power to express himself more accurately and more vividly as well.

If a similar remedy is given in too low a potency, I have learnt that another type of aggravation can happen. This, in my experience, can also be an intensity of symptoms, often accompanied by one or more keynote symptoms of the remedy itself, or a stubborn and intense new symptom that is accompanied by general improvement. There is normally some clue that makes you even more certain of the remedy, and if you are brave in such a circumstance, and if you feel after reading this book that the original potency chosen must have been too low, then go higher and see what happens. It is my guess that you will be pleasantly surprised.

# CASE NINETEEN
*Male*
*2 years old*

*(This is the case of a little boy who I have treated since birth. He was born wheezy and clingy with a sticky eye, at around the same time as his maternal grandfather passed away. His first remedy was Pulsatilla 200c, and he did very well on it. He subsequently received a dose of Medorrhinum and a dose of Lachesis for an acute. In July 2002, I was made aware of his eczema. I gave him Calcarea carbonica 200c at the time. In September 2002 he received Arsenicum album 200c for a rattling cough, and his eczema improved somewhat afterwards.)*

### 04.03.03

*He is waking up crying a lot. He has very bad eczema on his cheeks, they are very red, raw and fiery. He has eczema on his legs too, and scratches till it bleeds. It seems to bother him mostly at night. He is better if mum or dad lies with him. He is a bit panicky in bed at night, if awake and on his own, and he appears relieved when he sees the face of one of his parents.*

*Sometimes, mum will go to him and he'll want dad. He can cry for hours at these times until he gets dad. He needs a body next to him. His sister will do. He'll put an arm out at night to feel if there's someone there.*

*If he is slightly off-colour, he will run after mum or dad. He's very attached to his dad.*

*He is a very sociable chap. He will talk to anyone, though he won't always go to anyone. The minute his sister is home from the crèche, he follows her around. Otherwise, he's a bit of a bounder. 'Hello world, I'm here', type of thing.*

*He's not talking a huge amount. If someone is upset at home, he'll cuddle them. He calls all women 'mum'.*

*Up until nine months old, he was happy to go to anyone. He was cuddled a lot as a baby. He provided a lot of comfort.*

*He is very determined. Very mischievous. Will knock something off a table or snatch something and run. It's a game. He makes sure you are watching.*

*He is easy-going. Likes water a lot. Is enthusiastic. Falls over quite a bit. Is restless.*

*He developed his eczema within a few weeks of his birth and when he goes to stay at grandma's (without his parents), his eczema will get worse, though he is never upset about going there, nor is he upset at all during his stay.*

**Comment:** *he seemed very Sulphurish. He was into everything; with a 'Here I am world', attitude. But, needing someone to be with him at night does not suggest Sulphur, and neither is it characteristic of Sulphur to sometimes be fussy and obstinate about who he wants to be with him.*

*If he feels off colour, he will run to mum and dad, and be less independent during the day too.*

*He is sympathetic, although in the consulting room I do not see him as a Phosphorus type.*

*When his parents are away and he stays with grandma, his eczema is worse, though he is happy to be there.*

*Sankaran says of Magnesium carbonicum - 'In most Magnesium carbonicum patients there is a total repression – they feel that they should not make any demands on anyone, should not ask for help. In this way, they may seem independent. They seem not to need any care from others, and in fact can be quite caring.' He also says earlier on in the essay on Magnesium carbonicum : 'It is the state of an infant dependent on the mother for nourishment, care, security and support, but who has been abandoned by his parents.'*

*To me, this was the heart of the case, for here was a child who, when at home, is needy at night and sometimes insistent upon exactly who lies on the bed with him, and yet, when his parents are away he does not complain. He therefore, needs a remedy that can appear independent but deep down is not, and that remedy is Magnesium carbonicum. This was my assumption, and my gut feeling told me it was correct, but still I was not sure. I decided to give a low potency for that reason.*

**Prescription:** *Magnesium carbonicum 30c, daily for three days.*

**26.03.03**

*Very itchy. Skin has flared right up. Scratching loads and breaking the skin. His face is very bad.*

*He is very clingy and he has lost his appetite.*

*After Magnesium carboncium 30c, he insisted upon having the light on at night. At first he would cry for dad and then mum. He didn't know who he wanted.*

*He only wants fruit, and he wants it all the time. Melons and grapes especially.*

*He just wants mum or dad, and he can't bear someone leaving.*

*He is more grumpy than normal, if he doesn't get his own way. If he doesn't like what he hears, he will argue with his sister. He will take things from her and throw them away. Then he sits down and starts to scratch and cry. He will run to his sister if he is shouted at. He is scratching all the time, even in his sleep.*

*If he sleeps during the day, he wakes improved, but most of the time he fights sleep.*

*He's not interested in sweets.*

*There's an acrid discharge from his nose.*

**Comment:** *to me, this is a more exaggerated Magnesium carbonicum picture. Wanting fruit (2). Bad tempered. Sour/acrid discharges. Cannot bear to be left. The picture is more vivid. I am more sure the remedy is correct. I therefore decided to go up in potency and not having a 200c in stock, I went even higher, but just one dose to deal with the aggravation.*

**Prescription:** *Magnesium carbonicum 1M, sd(single dose).*

**08.04.03**

After Magnesium carbonicum 1M, there was a big difference. By the next day, he was back to his old self. That night he slept fairly well.

His skin has cleared a lot now. There is only a small patch on his right cheek and some on his legs.

He still wants a parent with him at night, but it's better. He's not so clingy.

**Comment:** I did not repeat the remedy at that point, but gave mum a dose of Magnesium carbonicum 1M to take away with her. My instructions were to give the remedy if his eczema started to deteriorate, or if in six to eight weeks time there has been no further improvement.

I often give remedies for my patients to hold on to if I think they might regress before I see them next time. One of my pet hates is having patients return after a long while, only to tell me that they started to get worse again soon after they saw me the last time. This is very irritating, especially if I had chosen not to repeat a remedy that had previously worked well, as I do dislike wasting time in any context.

I know it is controversial, but I am pretty sure that if a 'deep' remedy is chosen, and if the energy of the patient is fine, then the optimum potency is high.

'Deep' meaning one that resonates within the depths of the patient by mirroring the core of the problem.

**Therefore, if a patient aggravates in this circumstance after a remedy that is too low, it would be wise to go up in potency. For it is as if the lower potency has not got the energy to extinguish the problem in its entirety and as it tries to, it disturbs, and fizzles out.**

'For the purpose of effecting the cure, as the organism must be susceptible to the remedy, so the remedy must be susceptible to the organism and its concerning organs.....THE MORE SUSCEPTIBLE THE ORGANISM, THE HIGHER THE POTENCY AND THE FINER THE DOSE.'

FINCKE ON HIGH POTENCIES
PUBLISHED 1865

# SO IS AN AGGRAVATION REALLY NECESSARY?

In certain circumstances, I believe so, but not always. What I mean to say is, if the energy of the person is good and the clarity of the picture vivid, then an astute homeopath will probably recognise the remedy and give it in an appropriate potency. Usually this happens when the case is not too complicated and the vital force of the patient is pretty strong. In such a situation, I believe, an aggravation is not necessary.

Now, at the other end of the spectrum, you may come across low energy, many seemingly unconnected symptoms, a maintaining cause, and a patient who is in some way or even lots of ways, suppressed. Or a case where the homeopath needs to choose a remedy from a list of possibles. It is as if the case and probably the patient is mixed up. This suggests to me that an aggravation is probable, and should be welcomed as part of the healing process.

# POTENCY AND CASE-TAKING

Which brings me quite nicely to my next topic, that of potency and case-taking. What has case-taking got to do with potency selection? , I hear you ask. I do not categorically know, but I have this idea. Bear with me and I shall explain.

If potency is matched to energy in some way, then is not the energy in the consulting room important too? The energy of the prescriber? His/her ability to bring out certain aspects of the patient?

If the prescriber knows how to, and is used to guiding patients to seek their own depths, and the patient has revelations about himself in the consulting room that have not been gleaned before, then even before a remedy has been taken, the healing process must have begun, and the patient's energy increased in some way. The remedy chosen will then, more than likely, be fairly deep and the potency will probably be higher.

On the other hand, if the case-taking is superficial, the patient leaves the consulting room without having had his depths explored by his mind, so to speak. His awareness is therefore the same as before he had the consultation. No dynamic shift has taken place. The potency has not been raised by the consultation, and the remedy is more likely to be a superficial one too, making the most appropriate choice of potency lower.

What do you think?

# POTENCY, DOSAGE AND THE PRACTITIONER

If the above is true, then the practitioner might also want to look at his/her own miasmatic taint, as this will affect the potency he gives too. If, for example, the homeopath is very sycotic, then the temptation is to go in too high, and maybe even too often.

A psoric practitioner would more than likely underestimate the potency and dosage. A syphilitic prescriber... well let us hope there are not too many of those around! A tubercular homeopath might need to use different and unusual potencies, not wishing to be too restricted in his choices, and might change his mind often about what he thinks is correct. And just like Goldilocks when she finds baby bear's porridge, someone expressing the cancer miasm is going to get it just right, even if it kills him to do so!

# POTENCY AND THE CASE ITSELF

And of course, the case itself will dictate the potency. Sometimes, no matter how well you normally 'take the case', you will have a patient come in who tells you very little about themselves or their problem. You can sit there for hours and learn nothing more than a few snippets of information about them. These, then, are our most suppressed cases, and in my opinion need pretty low potencies, at least in the beginning, to gently draw them out over a period of time. If there is no pathology, and I am sure of what I want to give, I can go higher in such circumstances, say a 30c. If I am less sure, I will choose an LM. In a way, I suppose I do this to forcibly stimulate the energy of the person in order to provoke a response.

Conversely, other patients come in and give it to you on a plate. You almost get the feeling that they have swallowed a materia medica, so perfectly do they describe and act out their remedies. You are left in no doubt at all exactly what remedy they need right now. If someone like this comes to see me, and there is no pathology, they will always receive a high potency, say a 10M or even 50M, and I cannot remember one time when this has been a problem instead of a delight.

More commonly though, most patients fall somewhere between these two extremes, making 200c and 1M much used potencies in my practice. I give these potencies when I am pretty sure of the remedy, there is little or no pathology, and I am not too worried about anything at all that might make this potency inappropriate, for example, the patient being on medication.

# POTENCY AND ALLOPATHIC MEDICATION

In the early days, I used to think that allopathic medication would antidote the remedy or at least *might* antidote the remedy. I suppose to a certain extent, I still do worry about it whenever I give a prescription to someone taking ongoing conventional treatment.

I am trying to rack my brains to think of a case where I thought this might have happened. It is difficult, because if, by the time I see a person next, his remedy has not done something, then I tend to believe it is the wrong remedy, or these days the wrong potency of the right remedy. So, my mind just does not focus on the idea that a person's medication has interfered with the success of the prescription.

But because of my worry, I usually give an LM or a repeated low potency, just in case. I have also tried repeating higher potencies weekly. I did this a while back and abandoned the procedure. I am sure I must have done that because LMs and low potencies worked better.

If you think about it, that would make sense with my findings so far. Actually, being on allopathic medication is one of the most obvious forms of suppression there is, and suppression equals less clarity for the prescriber, something hidden, and in turn that equals a lower potency.

# NOT REALLY ABOUT POTENCY

I interviewed Ian Watson today and there is something I want to say. It is not really about potency, but I want to say it anyway. Ian has inspired me, and I want to take his lead.

As homeopaths, if we care and are passionate about our profession, then we want to get better at our craft. 'Better' means still learning and taking note of things when they happen.

As long as a homeopath does this, he/she is, even at the very beginning of his/her career, a good-enough homeopath: A homeopath on the road to competence via discovery. It is a road where none of us, even the greats, ever arrive. The journey takes forever, so forgive yourself for what you do not already know, and know that, if your intentions are honest about working with people to help them get stronger, then you are likely to do good along the way. And when you do not, be aware, and learn some more.

OK, preaching done.

# ENERGY

How strange! This is a book on potency and dosage of an energetic medicine, and it has taken me nearly one hundred pages before discussing the subject of energy at all. Well, the truth is, I think I actually might have avoided it.

I had this preconceived idea that this should be the most informative and most important part of this book, but it is not going to be, because I am not a scientist and do not understand essays and books full of scientific data that attempt to prove or disprove that homeopathy works.

I only have my training as a homeopath (including post-graduate training) and my clinical experience since I qualified, so all I know about energy is only that which I have been told and that which I have observed.

As you can see from the interviews, my comprehension of energy is something I have worked on. I am not sure if I understand it totally, but I have come to some conclusions based on what I have been told and what makes sense to me. Please understand that what I say next is my opinion. You may have a better explanation.

Firstly, all energy expressing a disease is warped energy. Energy, according to the dictionary is defined as:

*Intensity or vitality of action or expression; forcefulness.*

I understand, therefore, that a person's energy can be equated by how strongly they express themselves - how emphatically. Ideally, the force of the remedy should match the forcefulness of the problem. But what happens if you only match the intensity of the problem with the intensity of the potency and the remedy is not matched ideally enough?

In my experience, if this happens, then all that gets taken from that remedy by the vital force is energy. More energy is transferred to the body, enabling the patient to express themself more vividly. It appears that the energy becomes even more warped, but often there is more clarity, and this gives the homeopath a chance to improve on their choice of remedy. Imperfect remedies can do a little space-clearing, leaving the essence of the case bold and shining. I think, it is important to understand that the transferred energy, in itself, is a sign of greater, not lesser health. Therefore, greater clarity equals greater health, and more energy in the system equals greater health.

It is important to stress that intensity does not always bring clarity. I have certainly seen cases where there is lots of intensity, but at any one time you are only seeing part of the picture (SEE CHAPTERS ON PSYCHOSIS page 125 and HYPERSENSITIVITY page 124). These are energetic, but not healthy cases. In such a situation, you cannot afford to aggravate or throw more energy into the system if it is not going to cure. Here, I would suggest lower potencies, to take the energy down, so to speak, or a high potency of the simillimum if you know it from past case-taking.

If you bring the energy down, does that mean you are suppressing? In my understanding, no. Such cases need containing, and only when they are contained can the clarity come. They are the opposite of what we generally see, which is more energy equals more clarity. In these cases, the reverse is true, and lesser energy brings more clarity and therefore greater health.

If the forcefulness in the patient/problem is matched by too little energy, and the remedy does not fit at all closely enough you will probably get no reaction. Likewise, if the potency is too high and the remedy does not fit closely enough, you are likely not to get a reaction.

If the potency is too low and the remedy is good, you can still get no reaction. Although you are more likely to get some reaction; some movement towards the healing process. Maybe even a big movement towards the healing process. The vital force will ask you for a higher potency. It will either produce more symptoms that are not cured with time or the symptoms the patient had presented with are more intense or no longer abating with the original potency, or the remedy action is too short lived. In these cases it is as if the vital force is stirred but not stimulated enough for a perfect curative action (SEE CHAPTERS ON STRANGE DISCOVERIES pages 79 & 90).

If the remedy is good, but the potency is too high, once again you can experience nothing happening, but I think this is unlikely. The remedy action can be short lived (see Francis Treuherz interview). An intensity of symptoms occur. Here, it is as if the vital force is over-stimulated and needs to be less fuelled.

I guess energy, like everything else in the universe, is best when it is balanced.

# POTENCY AND PATHOLOGY

A large proportion of people who come to me exhibiting pathology are already on allopathic medication (SEE CHAPTER ON POTENCY AND ALLOPATHIC MEDICATION page 107). In a way, this is a blessing in disguise. I cannot imagine the chaos and anxiety in my life if most of them were not. You see (and I am not sure if my patients are representative of everybody's practice), very few of my patients would put up with not being able to function for too long, or with pain for that matter. And you know what, I sympathise with them.

At the Society of Homeopaths annual conference three years ago I was afflicted with the most terrible toothache. It was excruciating, and I tried with the help of some wonderful homeopaths to find a remedy that would resolve my problem. I waited patiently for the remedies to work, but come nightfall, I could not stand it anymore. I took painkillers in the end. So, you see, if I could not stand the pain and restriction on my life, then how could I expect one of my patients to put up with it? Personally, I never suggest an allopathic drug. What I do suggest is – keep your conventional medication to an absolute minimum. As far as I am concerned, this takes the urgency and emergency out of the equation, and it buys me time to do my job properly.

However, there are those who are not on medication, and there are urgent and emergency situations to deal with sometimes. For those not on medication, what I do in terms of potency, greatly depends upon the pathology I am dealing with. I am much more likely to give higher potencies these days for eczema, asthma, arthritis, Crohn's disease, colitis, mental pathology, MS, etc. All these diseases I have dealt with successfully with high potencies in the past, i.e healing reactions without terrible aggravations. The remedies were given in high potencies originally, because the picture of their disease was so vivid that it denied any other possibility of remedy choice. I have found it a very rewarding way to practice. And of course, when the clarity is not there, the choice of potency will be lower, the scale descending alongside worsening picture quality.

The one bone of contention to the above methodology of potency choice is cancer. Personally, most of the time I have had the opportunity to treat this disease, the conventional treatment also being received by the patient has overwhelmed the patient's vital force to such an extent that I find myself treating side-effects only. By the time the patient has recovered from one bout of chemotherapy or radiotherapy, it is time for the next bout. Unfortunately, their life force eventually wanes so much that the prescribing pictures become too vague, and the remedies impotent.

Dr Ramakrishnan, in his book about cancer consistently chooses the 200c potency to treat this very serious disease. He picks remedies that resemble the pathology together with a nosode, and gives one remedy at a time with repeated doses for a week, sometimes in water. He alternates remedies weekly. He gets excellent results.[12]

---

[12] *A Homeopathic Approach to Cancer* by Dr A.U. Ramakrishnan and Catherine R. Coulter

# TOXICITY

I never look at a patient and think 'Oh my God, they are so toxic', and for this reason the idea of toxicity doesn't seem to influence my choice of potency. I am much more inclined to think that their immune systems have been greatly compromised in a certain way. It is just the way my mind works.

I always tell people that their remedies can produce a detox affect, that they can get a symptom or symptoms that show the body is getting rid of something. I include headache, skin rash, a cold, a bit of diarrhoea and more frequent urination in a list of examples. I tell them that if this happens the effect will be transitory.

Some patients do experience these types of symptoms at the beginning of treatment, or after having been prescribed a particular remedy. These types of remedy reactions are not the type of aggravations I will prescribe on generally, and usually if one waits, the remedy proves to be curative. I cannot think of a case like this where greater health has not happened.

Personally, I never prescribe *Nux vomica* and *Sulphur* together as a detox. I have never found it particularly useful when I have. I have heard some homeopaths praise a 200c of each on the same day, and others advocate 6c of each daily for a week. As a prescriber, I do not like to waste time. I like to get stuck in as quickly as possible and get the ball rolling whichever way it will. The best indicated remedy usually does this. I feel most confident when I am mirroring the vital force itself.

# POTENCY AND HEALTH

Well, what is health exactly?  As homeopaths we must ask ourselves this question, because if we are not sure how to evaluate it, then how do we know that a patient is getting better?  We have Hering's Law of course, but is Hering's Law enough to help us decide?  What about in longstanding mental and emotional cases?  Do you always know if your remedies are helping the patient, or are you just shuffling about the remedy states?  Are you well enough yourself to evaluate what well is?

These are difficult questions.  In my practice, I try not to be arrogant. Just because I am treating somebody, it is not a certainty that their health will improve. There is an assumption sometimes, that just by visiting a homeopath and receiving a remedy, the patient will have benefited in some way.  Why?  Maybe what they had was a negative experience, and why should that improve their health?  Or is every experience a healing experience? I believe, that how we are with our patients is just as important as the remedy itself, because if we are not sensitive, then we can be just another brick in their wall, and that, in my book, will not be getting them better at all.

It is beyond the scope of this book to discuss this subject in the depth it so warrants, but I must say a few words. This is not so much a personal point of view, but a quest to be able to answer the question.  My ideas come from all over the place:  Patanjali's *Yoga Sutras*, many homeopaths who have come before me including Samuel Hahnemann, Kent, Rajan Sankaran, all my interviewees published herein, BKS Iyengar, my patients, Jung, my experience as a human being etc, ad infinitum.

So, all of these things are what I look for in follow-ups and what I hope the patient will achieve:

* More clarity of vision. Less delusion. More truth.
* Self-awareness, together with an ability to see what's going on all around.
* More self-expression. More confidence. Less fear to be ourselves
* Courage to make choices.
* Self-love and the ability to trust one's true instincts.
* The ability to love others.
* A balancing of sufficient energy.
* Making spaces in our lives to grow.
* Fluidity coupled with stability.
* The disappearance of pathology.
* The acknowledgement that joy and pain are both part of life.
* The shedding of one's coping structures while still being able to cope.
* Honesty.
* Strength of character.
* Energy.

I am sure I could go on. But what about potency and health? Some homeopaths work in the way that as a person's health improves the potency goes down. I can make a very good intellectual case for why this should be so. I could say that as the energy in a patient's pathology expires, so the energy in the remedy should diminish as well. But I have only done this once and it backfired on me (SEE CASE 18 page 94), so I tend not to practice this way.

For some reason, I have always done the opposite, believing that **as the patient becomes more healthy and therefore more energetic, he needs a higher potency. This has generally worked for me**, but what about Francis Trueherz case of needing to go down in potency, having been up really high, to get the remedy to work again (SEE INTERVIEW WITH FRANCIS TRUEHERZ page 181). As I write this, it has occurred to me that I have done this too. I have used an LM successfully, and when it was no longer curative, I gave a centesimal potency which worked for a while but did not seem as dynamic as the LM for this particular patient, so I went down to an LM again and the remedy was successful once more.

Why should this be so? For my patient, I suspect that the remedy was perhaps not the simillimum, and therefore I needed a better remedy in a higher potency perhaps. I do not know, but there must be an explanation.

Any ideas?

# ASCENDING POTENCIES

For the reasons described in the previous chapter, I usually increase the potency as the case progresses. If I change the remedy I usually think again about the potency I would like to use. My reasons for using a particular potency are based upon the clarity of the disease picture, as I have already stated many times in this book.

I know there are homeopaths who will give a 30c, 200c, and 1M of the same remedy in one prescription, but I am not one of these homeopaths and am therefore unqualified to comment on the usefulness of doing this. I believe that the reasoning behind three doses of a remedy in ascending potencies over a short period of time is to make the reaction of the 1M gentler, or to hedge ones bets.

I feel this way of prescribing is similar to giving two remedies at once because you are not sure which one is correct. Whenever I have done anything like this it always complicates the case management aspect, or what to do next. I like to keep things as simple as possible. For the most part, one remedy in one potency makes the decisions about follow-on prescriptions easy, and that is the way I like it. I also learn so much more if I prescribe in this way.

# DESCENDING POTENCIES

Let me confess here and now that I have done it. I have given patients who were not benefiting from single remedies, a series of remedies in descending potency in one prescription. The method I used is detailed in the book *Classical Homeopathy Revisited* by Jean Cole and Roger Dyson.

And was it useful. Not always, but in certain cases, yes. Some patients' health improved, others did not. None of them were 'cured'. It was desperate measures; when I really felt I had to do something and nothing else was working. None of the patients I treated this way were worse off because of it, but I still needed to find a remedy that was ultimately homeopathic to their case.

So, do I still use this method of prescribing? No. And why not? I guess, because it has been a long time since I have found myself in that desperate position of needing to do *something*. And would I do it again? I hope I will never feel that I need to.

For other ideas on descending potencies, see chapter on Potency and Health page 114.

# POTENCY AND MIASM

See Anthony Bickley interview

# LESSER USED POTENCIES

See interviews.

# POTENCY, DOSAGE AND ACUTES

As homeopaths, we tend to see prescribing for acutes in a different way to prescribing for a chronic complaint. We see acutes as high energy, fast moving, and we tend to give instructions to the patient to take the remedy more often than we would do if we have our eye on the chronic condition.

I was taught in the first year of college to use the potencies 6c, 30c or 200c to treat an acute. I understood that in acute circumstances, I should never go higher.

In the beginning years of my practice, I viewed acute outbreaks as completely separate entities from the chronic condition, and I prescribed mostly 30c's in the very early days and 200c's a bit later on, and I prescribed them routinely three to four times a day.

Mostly, this prescribing technique served me well. I automatically assumed that if the patient got better quickly, I had found a good remedy, and if they did not then the remedy was not a curative one.

These days, I see acutes a bit differently. Thanks to my discoveries about potency, I will change the potency to fit the problem (SEE CHAPTERS ON STRANGE DISCOVERIES pages 79 & 90). I now feel it can be appropriate to go much higher than a 200c, if the remedy picture is so vivid that it is screaming at me, and the intensity is there, I am happy to give a 10M, although I have rarely felt the necessity to go much higher than that.

I will also use dosage in a more fitting way. For example if the picture is unclear but the intensity is there, I will go low; a 6c or a 30c and repeat the remedy very often, anything from every ten minutes to hourly or two hourly depending on the case.

If the remedy is clear and it is a moderate case of urgency, then I usually give a 200c, three times a day. If the remedy is clear but the case needs to improve urgently, a 200c hourly, two hourly, three hourly, depending on the case.

I will use a 1M daily, usually only when the 200c has proved curative, but its power ran out of steam. But I do not usually give it often - three times over twenty four hours then review, or daily for a few days - tends to suffice.

If I give a 10M, it is usually daily for a few days and sometimes just one dose.

I have used LMs for acutes, where I think the patient needs the same remedy as they are already on, and if it is an LM, then I will up the dosage accordingly. Or if someone has been well for some time and they have an LM at home, then I tell them to take it.

If I start off an acute with one potency, and that works well initially, then does not any more, I will usually get the patient to plus (SEE CHAPTER ON PLUSSING REMEDIES page 65) the remedy before going up in potency. Often this works well.

# POTENCY, DOSAGE AND MAINTAINING CAUSES

Question: When does a modality become a maintaining cause?
Answer:   When it can be removed, and if removed the problem is then alleviated.

For some weeks now I have pondered upon this question, as to how maintaining causes affect dosage for the most part, and I have come to the conclusion that there are two different types of maintaining cause.

1)  The type of maintaining cause that poisons the system
e.g mercury in one's teeth, pollen during the hay fever season etc
2)  An emotional maintaining cause
e.g. a wicked family member, an over-stressful job etc

These two different types of maintaining cause seem to affect the need to repeat remedies differently.  The former type usually demands more frequent prescribing, especially when the reaction to an offending substance in the system is to produce an allergic reaction. I have found in this instance that **the remedy needs to be repeated often, sometimes three times a day while the allergen persists**. Conversely, I have also found that this need not necessarily be the case, and therefore a 'repeat remedy as needed' is good advice. Interestingly enough, I have found that it is not usually the offending substance itself that is prescribed in potency in these cases, but some other unrelated remedy, *Nux vomica* or *Natrum muriaticum* for hay-fever, for example.

**When the offending substance does not produce a typical allergic reaction, but other types of disease symptoms like thrush or mouth ulcers in the case of mercury poisoning, then I have found that I usually repeat the remedy for a number of days**, and after that it does not need to be repeated again for quite a while.

In the latter type of maintaining cause, I prescribe in the same way as if there is no maintaining cause. This type of maintaining cause does not seem to require more than a single dose of a high potency remedy (if that is the appropriate thing to do when assessing the rest of the case).

As far as potency is concerned, a maintaining cause in itself does not seem to affect my choice of potency.

# POTENCY, DOSAGE AND ANTIDOTING

Antidoting is something I have become more conscious of just recently. I was always fairly aware of allopathic medication somehow interfering with the remedy process, and for that reason, for a long time now, have almost routinely given LMs in a case where someone is taking medicine from the doctor on an ongoing basis.

But for most of my career I have pretty much pooh-poohed the idea that remedies can get antidoted. It just seemed so bizarre to me that this can happen. I mean if the remedy kick-starts a healing reaction by firing the vital force in some way, then how can a drink of coffee three days later, or cleaning your teeth with mint toothpaste, tell it No, do not do that, and turn the whole thing around again, like a bunch of workmen quitting on the job?

Perhaps, if the list of antidotes did not go on and on, I might have taken it on board, but as a student there were lecturers who would not treat patients on the Pill, others who taught us that cannabis and hash antidoted remedies, and in Samuel Hahnemann's the *Organon*, under aphorism 260, in footnote 140, there is an enormous list of foodstuffs that one must avoid if the remedies are to have a positive affect. I mean please, at this rate I was going to have to ask of my patients to have the strength of will of an ascetic and the lifestyle of a nun, and that is before they have even got started on their healing journey!

So, I adopted the attitude that the remedy will work anyway, despite an almost unavoidable, inhospitable environment.

In my formative years, I did not tell anyone about coffee and mint, and I treated everyone, from people who were on the Pill to marijuana junkies. I did however tell patients to take their remedies at least ten minutes either side of food and drink (I thought they could handle this one, as it is an instruction that applies to certain allopathic drugs and therefore what they are used to), but I also put remedies in food for my dog and my cat. Then I tried out eating and drinking after taking my remedies. Amazingly, I found out in that way that our remedies have more spunk than you would think, and for the most part they all get through!

I have always been pretty hot on telling people how to store remedies, and I store mine well; in a cool dark place away from strong smells, mobile phones, and any form of radiation. Do we need to do that? I do not know, but I am not taking the chance that my expensive and lovingly prepared remedies might get spoiled in some way, and anyway I have a great fondness and respect for my dispensary. It has helped a lot of people to get better and therefore deserves to be looked after!

However, I have learnt to take the antidoting factor into consideration if someone is not reacting at all to what I consider to be a good remedy, at least a good enough remedy to have created a stir, if not a mighty dynamic shift. I will always quiz a patient if this is happening. I will ask them about coffee and mint. I do give a leaflet with every first prescription that gives advice on how to take and store remedies, but I will also check at this point to see if they have heeded my advice.

I remember one elderly gentleman was drinking decaffinated coffee (coffee is a reported antidote for his particular remedy)[13] and when he stopped, he started to respond to *Psorinum* LM1. I also treated another lady who started to respond to her remedy after giving up coffee. These are isolated cases. In my experience most remedies do not get antidoted.

I must say that the majority of people who seem to 'antidote' their remedies are people who know quite a lot about homeopathy, and claim they have gone backwards since that cup of coffee that they did not mean to drink etc., and in these instances I often wonder if we create our own reality.

Should we perhaps give different instructions for everyone based on their remedy? For example, should we tell all *Psorinum*'s about coffee, all *Lac defloratum*'s about milk, all *Nux vomica*'s about alcohol, rich food and drugs? But what worries me is, what happens when these people are hooked on some thing or some lifestyle; does that make them untreatable? In my book no, not in my experience. So find a better remedy, or find a more appropriate potency, because the remedies work in spite of a person's self abuse, and if the remedies are well chosen, then their habits should diminish or they should gain the strength to conquer them in some way. After all, isn't that all part of the process of cure?

---

[13] See Boericke's Materia Medica chapter on *Psorinum.*

# POTENCY AND AGE

In my opinion, age is not a criterion for selecting a certain potency, but it is something to be considered. I believe that the vital force of the person will indicate the choice of potency each and every time.

In the same way that the character and expression of the vital force will indicate which remedy, so the forcefulness and clarity of that expression will indicate the relevant potency in ways already described in this book.

But having said that, age is definitely a factor that one can take into account. I think that, as a prescriber, pulling oneself up short and saying 'Now hold on a minute this person is eighty-five do I really want to prescribe a 10M? Is like your computer asking you 'Do you really want to save this?, it just gives you the option to think again and therefore to avoid making a careless mistake.


# POTENCY AND ENERGY OF THE PERSON OR ENERGY OF THE DISEASE?

If the vital force is exhibiting a lot of energy in the pathology, but the patient's energy resources are sapped of energy, and the picture is crystal clear, then I would give a potency that mirrors the energy of the state. If the remedy was screaming at me, I would go in with a high potency.

If, however, I was prescribing for the person in a constitutional way, because even though the symptoms are dramatic they are in themselves inconclusive remedy-wise, and the patient has little energy, then I would go in with a low potency, a potency that is homeopathic to the energy of the state that I am treating.

In this way **I always prescribe a potency that corresponds with the energy I am treating at the time**.

# POTENCY AND HYPERSENSITIVITY

Hypersensitive people are the loose cannons of the homeopathy world. They are notoriously difficult to treat because they are sensitive to everything and things are consistently changing, and not, it seems, for the better. They do not walk into our practices often, but when they come, they seldom stay, and in true characteristic fashion they move quickly on to the next thing and the next thing and the next...

They are almost the opposite of the sycotic miasm, where things are fixed, and yet they are the same. For these people things are moving fast, but they are hidden too. They are slippery and fall through our grasp, because just when we think we have found their true remedy, they are proving something else and off they go on another tangent.

As you can see if you read through part two of this book, one of the questions I have almost consistently asked is, do you have any advice to give on hypersensitive patients?

From my perspective, I have observed that they certainly have energy and fluidity, but no stability. I think what happens with these patients is that we tend to look at them in a tunnel-visioned way. We need to be able to stand back and ask ourselves, 'Hold on a minute, what is really going on here?', before we give the next remedy.

I guess, in general we are looking at a box of remedies like *Mercury*, *Thuja*, *Phosphorous*, all the plants, etc., and until we are really sure that we are matching them correctly, then lower potencies are called for in my opinion.

I have two patients who are pretty sensitive to remedies. I am not going to present their cases here because there is little to be gleaned by doing so. But, I have noticed over the years of prescribing for them that they do not need much of a remedy to get things moving. **Low potencies and infrequent doses even in acutes seems to be the most effective.**

# POTENCY AND PSYCHOSIS

I view psychosis in a similar way to hypersensitivity when it comes to potency. Things can appear incredibly vivid, but what you are seeing at any one moment is just a very small part of the whole.

I have one patient who responded very well to an LM of *Veratrum album* when he was going through a psychotic episode. I actually met him in an acute phase of his illness and things appeared to indicate that remedy at the time. As I got to know him better, it turned out that his bigger picture spelled out the remedy *Aurum*. These two remedies seem worlds apart I know, but as Rajan Sankaran states in his book *The Soul of Remedies,* 'Aurum people are highly moralistic, principled and orthodox. However, sometimes it can work the other way round, i.e. finding the task too high; *Aurum* becomes then irresponsible and immoral'. This is what happened to my patient. I think a higher potency of *Veratrum album* at the time, might have exacerbated a critical situation even more.

In another case of acute psychosis, in which I did not prescribe as honourably or successfully, I took each new delusion that the patient expressed and tried to prescribe for it, thinking erroneously each time that I now had the central delusion of the case. The sort of potencies I used were 30c and 200c, but as you can imagine, I got into an awful pickle with it. The patient ended up in hospital. It was not until I stood back from the shifting sands of the acute episode and viewed the bigger picture that I realised what remedy the patient really needed.

**I really can not stress enough that in my experience of acute psychosis you really do have to see the bigger picture or truly understand what the vital force is trying to tell you in order to use even moderately high potencies successfully.** Relatives can be extremely helpful in these situations to throw a bigger light on the situation, but failing that I have found that a low potency, like 6c, maybe 12cs , or LM, are really your best bet for a gentler reaction.

# HYPERACTIVITY, ADD AND ADHD

I would have thought the same rules apply to hyperactivity and ADD/ADHD as they do to psychosis and hypersensitivity, when it comes to potency.  **But on reflection when treating hyperactivity and ADD/ADHD, I have definitely had distressed parents phone me up after just a few doses of an LM, and cannot remember a time when the reaction from a centesimal produced that big a reaction.  Having said that, I have also treated a boy incredibly successfully and painlessly, without having to go higher than *Tuberculinum* LM1.**

With hyperactivity and ADD/ADHD it is usually a case of the remedy working or not working. And in children, hyperactive behaviour and ADD/ADHD is difficult to shift.  I have found that when these kids are unwell they respond to the remedies nicely, but in quite a few cases, have been stubborn when it comes to trying to balance them mentally.  The successes I have had in this field are mostly because parents have persisted with the treatment through all its ups and downs.  Many give up too early and do not give it enough of a chance.

One of my most successful cases to date is a boy who was really quite bad, but as far as his mum was concerned always responded well to his remedies, though I never saw the improvement in him until quite late into the treatment.  He would do well on a remedy, then either revert to worse behaviour, or she would simply have had enough of him and bring him back in desperation for a homeopathic remedy to help.

It took about two years to get him to the point where he had stopped trying to destroy all the toys in the consulting room.  I started treating him with LMs, changing his remedy often as more elements of his personality were revealed to me. On looking back at his case, I noticed that I used low to middling potencies throughout, because there was never a prescription that I felt encapsulated his whole picture.  Nevertheless, when I take an overview, I do think that he grew more and more comfortable in his own skin, and therefore did very well on the remedies.

The above case is quite typical of how I have found hyperactive/ADD/ADHD patients respond to homeopathic treatment, and using potency in the above way seemed to prove the most successful when compared to other modus operandi.

# POTENCY AND THE HEALING PROCESS

I suppose, one way of telling how healthy your patient is, is to look at the potencies that you are prescribing. Higher potencies meaning that the vital force has the energy to express itself and the ability to be clear with the messages it is sending out.  To me, this is an expression of a healthy vital force.  Therefore, if you are prescribing high potencies for your patients then they are pretty healthy, conversely low potencies would mean an expression of ill health.  If the potencies that you are using are ascending, then you must be getting somewhere. If they are descending and you are becoming more and more flummoxed, it Is time to ask yourself if your input has aided or hindered the flow of expression from the vital force.

Of course, once the simillimum is found, and the patient's problems start to fade, then whether you decide to descend or ascend the potency seems to be a bit of a bone of contention amongst homeopaths. **The ascending scale seems to work best for me as long as the appropriate remedy remains the same.**

# DOSAGE AND SPEED

I think that as far as dosage goes, speed is one criterion.  **If, for instance, an ailment is moving fast, as in an acute, then more frequent doses of the remedy become necessary** (unless the nature of the problem is incredibly vivid too, when a few high doses of the simillimum is probably all you need). Conversely, if a disease has been very slowly getting worse over a number of years, then less frequent doses are more appropriate (if you are using moderate or high potencies).

**There is also a feeling, that the more fixed a person or problem is, the more doses they are going to need to kick the vital force into action.** Conversely, the more moveable, impressionable, and malleable a person/problem is, the fewer doses they need to get the healing process flowing. **In terms of potency, I would be looking at a lower potency for a fixed state and a higher potency for the opposite situation.**

How long should a homeopath or patient wait before the effect of a remedy becomes apparent?   Well, I always ask patients what happened after they took their remedy.  Most people report that a discernible affect from the remedy is pretty much immediate, or at least noticeable after two to three days. It is unusual but not unheard of, for people to report no change for two weeks,

My most outstanding case to date is a little boy who was given a single dose of *Belladonna* 200c for eczema and asked to return after four weeks.  His mum cancelled the appointment because the family were going away on holiday, and rebooked the follow up for seven weeks after the initial consultation.  At the follow-up mum reported that the eczema had remained the same for six weeks and now had completely disappeared.  I did wonder about the holiday being an ameliorating factor, but it was about a year later when I saw him again with a slight return of his old problem.

# CHANGING POTENCY

I can see three reasons for changing the potency:

The first is because a remedy has proved successful, the picture remains the same and you have no reason to change the remedy, but the remedy no longer stimulates the healing process in that potency. I normally go up in potency when this happens (BUT ALSO SEE CHAPTERS ON ASCENDING AND DESCENDING POTENCIES pages 116 & 117).

The second reason is because the remedy in that potency did not work at all, but you are almost one hundred per cent positive that you have the correct remedy. I can go either up or down in potency when this happens (SEE CHAPTERS ON STRANGE DISCOVERIES pages 79 & 90).

Thirdly, the remedy has aggravated and you feel the necessity to prescribe, but you do not feel it is appropriate to change the remedy. I can go up or down in potency when this happens, once again see chapters on strange discoveries.

If the duration of the remedy is too short, then I will consider changing the potency, but might not necessarily do so. I will definitely look over the case again to make sure I am doing the best I can remedy-wise. Usually, if this happens and I do not wish to change the remedy, sooner or later I will have to change the potency anyway because that potency will no longer kick-start the vital force into healing.

These days, I make it my policy not to change the potency if the previous dose of the remedy has acted with only positive results and does not need to be repeated too often.

# DOSAGE

Now that I have said everything I have wanted to say about potency, I would like to say a few words about dosage.

Firstly, I come from the school of thought that believes one dose can be a single granule or a whole bottle, it is still one dose, and it is the repeating of a remedy that constitutes a dose and needs to be taken into account. I guess I think this way because it seems logical to me that we are transferring energy to the patient via the remedy. The amount of energy is contained in the potency. It is as if we are sending a message, and the same message is transferred no matter what the surface area of the messenger.

The way I think could easily be wrong. Just because the above seems to make sense to me does not make it right. After all, many allopaths discard homeopathy on the grounds that it does not make sense. But based on my beliefs, I do not tend to give significance to the messenger; the pill. I do not tend to buy smaller and larger pillules to modify the dose, and I rarely give two or more pills (and if I do it is because two dropped into the cap instead of one and I lazily gave them). By the same token I am never exact about how many drops or spoonfuls of liquid my patients should take on their tongue. Nothing that has ever happened so far has made me think that this is not a sensible way to practice.

Yet I am open to the suggestion that this is because I have not paid enough attention to this area of dosage; that in fact there were lessons to learn, but they were not apparent enough for me to notice. I have certainly had patients who have sworn that two drops of an LM had a lesser impact than three for example, but they modified their drops to suit their own needs. None of these patients reported anything too uncomfortable and such patients have been few and far between.

Still, some of the homeopaths I interviewed have paid great attention to the messenger. They have observed things like liquids being gentler than solids, olfacation being stronger than either liquids or solids, and two pillules being stronger than one.

As far as chronic cases and the higher centesimal potencies go (30c and upwards), another aspect of dosage that is really interesting is, is there any difference between the single dose and the collective single dose i.e one pillule a day for three days (as I tend to prescribe), or three pillules over twenty four hours, versus one single pillule?

My rationale for the way I practise is, rightly or wrongly, to give one a day for three days just in case one does not get through, or is antidoted at source in some way, and the odds are that all three doses will not be. But is this folly? I am starting to give just one single dose more often now, especially in cases where I worry about aggravation. So far, I have been impressed and happy with the outcome whenever I have prescribed in this way. My feeling is that sometimes the three doses can be more of an irritant to the patient than just one, and at other times it really does not matter at all. I guess what I try to gauge is how fixed or how easily malleable do these people appear. If I gauge them to be very fixed than I repeat it daily for up to five days and if I gauge the opposite then a single dose suffices.

By the same token, I have also started to give remedies weekly to people I suspect might need their remedy to be repeated more often, and this method has proved incredibly successful some of the time and downright confusing at others.

To illustrate this, I had a case just recently, where I was treating a little boy for emotional/behavioural problems with *Lycopodium* 200c I asked mum to administer one pill weekly. During the follow-up consultation, she reported that when they were on holiday, they forgot to take the remedy with them and the child went for two weeks without a dose of his remedy. She said that by the time they came home his problem had accelerated again, after abating somewhat when he took the first dose. She said within hours of taking the second dose he had begun to calm down. My reaction was to up the potency to 1M when his behaviour reverts next time, in anticipation that it might do so before I was to see him again. In that case I was very pleased to have given the remedy weekly, and things would not have gone so swimmingly if I had not.

Other cases where I have used this method of dosage have left me with a dilemma. The dilemma is, if I have been prescribing weekly for some time, and things were working well, and then after a long while the patient gets worse again, do I stop the remedy? Have too many doses pushed the patient into a proving? Or do I need to go up in potency? What I choose to do in such an instance, is to stop the remedy first, then if the vital force does not balance itself out a bit within days, I will choose to go up in potency. This ambiguous situation does not arise if a single dose is prescribed.

Anyway, for me, the above rules mostly apply to higher centesimal potencies (30c and upwards) and when prescribing for a chronic layer of a case. I tend to routinely prescribe lower potencies more often for a chronic layer: two to three times a day for a tissue salt up to a 6c and daily for a 12c, and that works fairly well. I have already discussed dosage and LMs in the chapter on LMs, page 49.

**I think it is fair to say that the positive effects from higher potencies generally last longer than the positive effects from lower potencies, meaning that high potencies need to be repeated less often. However, sensitive patients can need only one dose of a 6c to initiate a healing response that will last a long time.**

As for acutes and dosage, please refer to a previous chapter in this book entitled Potency, Dosage and Acutes, page 118.

# DEPTHS AND LAYERS

Personally speaking, the only layers that I recognise are the constitution of the person to including the miasmatic taint and the problem or problems which may or may not echo the same remedy.

The vital force dictates what is to be addressed by the force and clarity of its expression at any one time, and by bringing characteristic symptoms to the fore that mirror a particular remedy. Sometimes a remedy can be a simillimum of the moment. What I mean is, sometimes a remedy can eradicate a recent problem that it mirrored exactly, only to reveal another remedy and problem that has been going on much longer, and which makes the problem you have just treated look like a spin-off of the complaint you are now treating.

But as far as potency and dosage goes, it does not much matter whether you are prescribing for a layer, the whole problem, or the constitution. What does matter is how accurately you match the remedy to what is uppermost in the case. The more accurate you are with your prescribing, the higher the potency should be. A homeopath's only measure of accuracy must therefore be how sure they are of the remedy they are prescribing. I believe you are more likely to get a better reaction from a partial match with a lower potency.

So, if you like, a deep remedy is a clear and accurate remedy, and conversely a partial match is a superficial remedy. An unsure match might be either but should be treated as superficial until symptoms are revealed that make you more certain. And in this way, **the deeper the remedy, the higher the potency should be. The more superficial the remedy, the lower the potency should be.**

# POTENCY AND THE 'WHAT I HAVE GOT IN STOCK' METHOD

There are times when I have had, what I consider to be an inappropriate potency in stock of a remedy that I have wanted to prescribe.  There are times when I have used that inappropriate potency and it has been as if the gods were shining down on me.

There have also been times when I have used the potency that I have had in stock and regretted it.  **I guess if you choose to gamble, some you win, and some you must lose.**

# POTENCY, DOSAGE AND PROPHYLACTICS

**When it comes to prophylactics, I always use 30c, which I suggest the patient takes one day before travel and weekly for as long as they are in suspected territory**. I do this because I am never quite sure how long the vital force retains the message. Therefore, I do not offer parents an alternative to childhood vaccinations etc.,. I do worry, however, about doing this for longer than two to three weeks, as I do not wish the traveller to incur proving symptoms either. I often couple this advice with ten drops of *Chelidonium* tincture, taken daily in fruit juice or water to tone the liver during their trip.

I also recently phoned Helios, Nelson's and Ainsworth's, to see what they advise over the counter in respect of prophylactics. Nelson's reported to me that they do not give such advice but would refer on to a homeopath. Helios and Ainsworth's advice was not a million miles away from mine. Helios recommends the 30c potency, mostly, too, and for most nosodes they suggest a weekly dose whilst abroad. They make an exception for malaria, which they suggest should be taken one week before travel and for four weeks after the traveller returns. So it seems they do not worry about proving symptoms at all. Sometimes for malaria prophylaxis they suggest *Natrum muriaticum* 6x and *Chininum sulphuricum* 6x daily.

Ainsworth's also use 30c potency and their advice is similar. They suggest that the traveller takes three doses in one day and repeat this weekly, or step up the dose to daily if the traveller comes into contact with an infected case. For malaria they suggest you take the remedy for one week before and three weeks after return, though they believed this was unnecessary. They informed me that they have an anti-cold and flu preparation which they suggest should be taken, one tablet on a Sunday and repeat every two weeks throughout the season. Last, but not least, prophylaxis for dog and cat ailments in homeopathic potency, which they suggest is administered daily for one week, then weekly for six weeks and then monthly for six months. And so it seems, that they too do not worry about proving symptoms.

Personally, I can prescribe prophylactically in other situations too. When I know that someone gets a skin rash from being in the sun, I have been known to prescribe *Sol* 30c, three doses before travel and to repeat only if it has some value and then runs out of steam. Likewise, I will prescribe *Caladium* for a person who gets bitten a lot by bugs or mosquitoes, in exactly the same way. *Arnica* for jet lag; I suggest *Arnica* 30c one dose before travel and one on arrival. For head lice, I usually give three doses of *Staphysagria* 200c; a higher dose because in this situation the patient is usually coming into direct contact with the contaminant.

In other situations, I will prescribe remedies in advance, if not prophylactically. For example, before dental work, before an operation, and for anticipatory fear. In all these situations I usually prescribe a 200c of the remedy or remedies that I suspect the patient is going to need. As for dosage, I will prescribe one dose beforehand and to be repeated daily after the event for as long as the remedy is appropriate and needed.

# WHAT TO DO IF.......

# YOU NEED TO CHOOSE A POTENCY

## Ask yourself these questions:

How positive are you that the remedy is chosen correctly?

If the answer is very, then choose a very high potency (1M, 10M and above)
If the answer is not at all, then choose a very low potency (6c , LM, 12c)
If the answer is pretty sure, but not certain, then choose a medium potency (30c, 200c)

On what basis are you giving the remedy?

If the answer is constitutional prescribing, then does the remedy also mirror the presenting complaint?

If the answer is yes, then go higher in potency.  If the answer is no, then go lower.

Do the patient's words mirror the patient's actions?

If yes, then go higher.  If no, then go lower.

Do you have a deep understanding of the case?

If so, then choose a higher potency.

Or is your understanding of the case 'superficial'?

Then choose a lower potency.

## How do you tell if you are prescribing 'superficially'?

If you are prescribing on any of these factors alone:

1. Totality of symptoms
2. Aetiology
3. Keynotes
4. Because the remedy is famous for a particular disease
5. Because the remedy has an affinity for a particular organ
6. A nosode to address a particular miasmic taint

Then your prescribing is superficial.

## Do any of the following circumstances appear in your case?

1. Is the patient or their symptoms suppressed?
2. Is the patient on allopathic medicine?
3. Is the person old?
4. Is the patient hypersensitive?
5. Does this patient psychologically need the support of more frequent Doses?

If so, you might want to think about giving a lower potency.

Choose:

6x      If you are looking at a very small part of a developed photograph. The image is clear.

6c      If you are looking at a negative of a photograph and you can just about make out some characteristics.

30c     If you are looking at a negative of a photograph and the image is quite clear but you know that when it has been printed this might change your perception.

200c  If you are looking at a printed photograph. The main subject is quite clear, but there are things in the background that you just cannot make out.

1M      The image is clear, but not sharp and just a little out of focus.

10M    The picture is screaming at you with life and vitality in full focus.

# YOU NEED TO CHOOSE A DOSAGE

Ideally, a remedy is repeated every time the previous dose no longer promotes a curative action, and this goes on until the remedy in the potency you are using no longer initiates a healing response.

## Ask yourself these questions:

How high is the potency I have chosen?

The higher your choice of potency, the less often the remedy should need to be given.

Here is a rough guide:

| For chronic complaints: | 6x and 6c | twice or three times daily |
| | 12c | daily |
| | 30c upwards | single dose, or split dose, then review after one month |
| | LM | daily |

| For acute complaints: | lower potencies | up to hourly |
| | middling potencies | up to six times in one day |
| | higher potencies | up to daily |

Reduce the doses in acute circumstances as the patient's health improves.

How obstinate/malleable do I think this patient's vital force will be?

Obstinate will indicate a call for more frequent repetition of the remedy. Malleable will indicate the need for less frequent doses.


How fast is the problem progressing?

Greater velocity needs to be matched with more frequent doses of the remedy. Conversely, a slow moving disease needs fewer doses of the remedy.


Is there a maintaining cause, and what type of maintaining cause is it?

A maintaining cause such as an allergen is likely to need more frequent prescribing.


Is the patient on allopathic medication?

If yes, then you may consider more frequent doses.

# YOUR PATIENT HAS AGGRAVATED

## Ask yourself these questions:

### Is the potency I have given too high?

Look at the case again. Ask yourself if you have overestimated your understanding of the case. If you think you have and you are following the guidelines set out in this book, then the potency you have given is too high.

At this point you can either give a lower potency. 6c is usually the preferred potency at this stage, or you can re-take the case to try and give an acute remedy for the aggravation or a better indicated remedy. Or, if the aggravation is not limiting the patient's daily life, then you can choose to wait.

### Is the potency I have given too low?

If the patient's symptoms are making you feel more and more certain of the chosen remedy, then the probability is that you have prescribed too low in potency.

At this point you will do well to go higher. Or, once again if the aggravation is not too intense then you can choose to wait.

### Has the remedy been repeated too frequently?

If the patient is taking his remedy often, then first of all stop it completely if an aggravation occurs. Wait till some time has elapsed, then either reduce the dosage of the original remedy by estimating how much of the medication his/her vital force is likely to need without tipping them into overload. Or wait until you see them next time before you re-introduce the prescription. Or treat the symptoms that have emerged by re-taking the case.

# AND WHAT DO I DO NOW?

The remedy has encouraged an 'acute' in the patient.

You can take the acute case and prescribe the indicated remedy, or you can encourage the patient to wait. But if the symptoms are severe, constant monitoring is required. It goes without saying that you must never be negligent.


Everything seems to have changed since the remedy.

Re-take the case and prescribe the indicated remedy in the appropriate dosage. If the remedy is unclear then prescribe low or decide to wait.


One month has gone by, and there is no sign of an amelioration.

Re-take the case. I would say your choice of prescription is close but not close enough. You have probably given the wrong remedy, but if you are still certain that your choice was perfect, then you could always try changing the potency.


The patient is proving to be hypersensitive to every remedy.

Prescribe low and infrequently.

# THE INTERVIEWS

*It was my intention when I started to write this book that all the findings on the previous pages would be solely my own discoveries.*

*However, it would not be fair not to mention that as these following interviews were conducted at different stages of my work, my questioning was often influenced by this, and the answers I received did sometimes help me to solidify my own thoughts.*

*Still, I hope it is reflected herein, that I have tried in earnest not to interpret (and therefore maybe wrongly interpret), nor claim for my own, the experiences of others. It is for this reason that these enlightening interviews appear here with the as little editing as possible.*

# Anthony Bickley

**MS:**   My first question is how do you select a potency?

**AB:**   I do a little schema for myself. I think about what the effect has been on the patient's vital force and what is the depth and speed of penetration into the vital force, and whether there is a particular maintaining cause. Then I look at the nature of the miasm and the nature of the remedy. All of those things will influence the choice of potency.

**MS:**   You refer to the depth of penetration of the vital force. Do you mean how strongly the problem has got hold of the patient?

**AB:**   How serious in homeopathic terms the case is. So, for example, if the patient has come to you with a burning desire to expose themselves on Tower Bridge, it is worse than if they have got a problem like an in-growing toe-nail. It penetrates deeper into the body's economy.

**MS:**   I assume when you have a very deep case e.g. of a man who wants to expose himself in full view of everybody, then you would go higher in potency, is that right?

**AB:**   Generally speaking higher, as long as you use the word higher rather than high.

**MS:**   How would a maintaining cause, for example, influence your choice of potency?

**AB:**   It would depend on the nature of the maintaining cause, of course. If there is a maintaining cause of a situational nature then obviously we have to follow Hahnemann and see what we can do about changing the maintaining cause, but the maintaining cause itself is actually going to make life more difficult for whatever remedy, potency, combination you have. So one needs to try and overcome the situation. You have to create a marginally stronger artificial disease and with a maintaining cause that usually means a more frequent repetition of the dose of a higher potency.

**MS:**   And the nature of the miasm, how would that effect the potency?

**AB:**   With the psoric miasm generally patients underfunction, and they need a bigger kick to get them started. Therefore, remedies which are psoric and patients who are psoric generally need more effort to get them moving. I am going to consider either using a higher potency or a bigger dose. I usually use a higher potency to start with. If using a psoric remedy, I would tend towards the upper scales rather than the lower.

**MS:**   And the nature of the remedy?

**AB:**   Well, the nature of the remedy within a miasm is that some remedies are totally psoric in the sense that they are totally underfunctioning, so they would need the very highest kicks. I rarely use *Psorinum* lower than 10M. *Sulphur* is a more active remedy than *Psorinum*, though it is still psoric to a large extent, and so I would often use Sulphur from 50c upwards, because there is a different scale of activity within the general miasm, and then they need a different scale of potency.

**MS:**   You use *Psorinum* very high because the essence is underfunctioning, so would that mean that with the remedy *Medorrhinum*, where the tendency is to over produce, you would use a lower potency?

**AB:**   Yes. Then of course when we come to *Syphilinum*, which works differently, because people who need this remedy react either very high or very low, but not very much in the middle.

**MS:** And *Carcinosin*?

**AB:** Well, I do not consider *Carcinosin* in this sense because there are only three things that can actually go wrong with the body. It can underfunction, it can overfunction, or it can function wrongly. So because we are talking about simple constructs here we do not need to look at that. *Carcinosin* itself, both as a remedy and as a miasm or taint, is generally deep-acting, and its effects take a little time to come out. When the symptoms do appear they are quite strong, so we tend to need medium ranges of potency.

**MS:** What would make you want to change a potency?

**AB:** Are we talking about follow-ups at this stage? Well it depends on whether the patient is more or less sick than they were when they started. So if I have given a remedy and the patient is less sick than they were previously, I would be giving them a lower potency.

**MS:** Do you have any information to share about aggravations that have not been documented before?

**AB:** Probably not. I am not a big believer in aggravations. I do not expect my patients to have aggravations. That does not mean they never have them, but the number of serious aggravations in twenty-five years could be counted on the fingers of one hand.

**MS:** If a patient has aggravated, do you prescribe or wait?

**AB:** That depends upon the nature of the aggravation and the nature of the patient. If it was a sign that something was seriously wrong rather than the body not being able to cope with the degree of kick I had given it, then I would of course want to prescribe. I would not necessarily have got the potency wrong, but there would have been something wrong with the prescription as a whole: therefore I would be prescribing. If, on the other hand, the aggravation is simply because everything is working very well, although the patient is having trouble coping, and encouraging them no longer works, so that they say, "I am going to go and take the antibiotic unless...", then I might prescribe on the aggravation, provided we have got the aggravating symptoms clear enough. After all, it is just an expression of the vital force like anything else.

**MS:** Supposing you have an aggravation and the symptoms are the same but less intense, and obviously at that point you are pretty sure of your remedy, and the patient is driving you mad, what do you do then?

**AB:** I put on my most emollient face and voice and encourage them and tell them to ring me tomorrow and the next day and the next day. Because I obviously want to do as little as possible while it is getting better.

**MS:** You never use a lower potency - or some people say a higher potency - to take the edge off the aggravation?

**AB:** I do not change the potency if things are doing well, if I can possibly avoid it. Every time I make a prescription I did not really want to make, something goes wrong and I regret it. I still regret some of the prescriptions I did make but that is not the point. When I know I should not do something and I still do it;,I always wish I had not.

**MS:** If you have an aggravation and you decide that you would like to wait, how long do you wait? In my experience sometimes aggravations do not lead to cure.

**AB:** Oh indeed, but if aggravations do not lead to cure they either give you more symptoms of the same remedy, accessory symptoms, so in that case you have probably got the remedy right but the potency or dose wrong, and then you will need to amend it. Or they will give you a new symptom which when you add it to the totality will indicate a different remedy.

**MS:** So what are your views on dosage?

**AB:** My view is that dosage matters, but not to everybody. It matters mostly to sycotic individuals, in the sense that sycotic individuals often need a very much smaller dose than anybody else. Then to the opposite scale, psoric individuals often need a bigger dose. I very often give my remedies in liquid form, but if I were giving pills then I might very well give two pills to a psoric patient and half a pill, or the equivalent, to a sycotic patient.

**MS:** Would you wait until they saw you next time before you repeated it?

**AB:** I have not got time to go into that in great detail, except I have got a whole schema which I use to explain this. But as a general rule, one prescription, or one dose in these circumstances, is usually enough. More does not necessarily mean better, but nor does it necessarily do harm. So my tendency is to give a single prescription in chronic cases. In acute cases there are a different set of rules that apply.

**MS:** Do you ever use LMs or plus remedies?

**AB:** Yes to both.

**MS:** And in what circumstances would you choose to do that?

**AB:** I usually use LMs in sycotic cases and in the more aggressively active syphilitic cases. I use LMs in single doses so I will give a single test dose and observe the reaction. I will want the patient to contact me in three or four days. If there has been no further reaction to the remedy, I will tell them to take two doses usually; one that day and one the next day, and to contact me in a further three days. If there has been no reaction, then I would expect them to actually take the LM for a week. That does not usually happen. Mostly they will react with either the single dose or one of the second doses.

**MS:** So you would use LMs almost in the same way as people use the centesimal scale?

**AB:** Yes.

**MS:** Do you have any information to share about sensitive people. For instance, do you have your own way of recognising sensitive people before you prescribe for them?

**AB:** Only by the nature of the symptoms and the discussion that you have with them. You are normally talking with the patient about how they react to situations and to ailments and what the degree of severity of their symptoms is and in those circumstances you look at that, the speed of the reactivity, the severity of the reactivity and then in conjunction again with whether they tend to overfunction, or wrongly function. If they overfunction, if they function wrongly, in an extreme manner, then they are likely to be more sensitive. So if that is the case I would be reducing the dose, I would be reducing the potency and I would probably be diluting the dose as well. That would be the case if I was thinking of using a centesimal or an LM.

**MS:** So you find if you dilute the dose it makes it gentler?

**AB:** If I dilute the dose then it is gentler.

**MS:** Do you have any questions on potency and dosage that you would like answered?

**AB:** I feel very comfortable with potency and dose. The only thing that bothers me is that people feel the need to make somebody else wrong. I do not feel the need to do this. I have a system which seems to work quite well and I have spent an amount of time with my students saying this is a system that I use, but I could also explain to you why other people's systems seem to work. I have not got time to go through that, but I think we need to stop being so precious about our own systems and just put them out there and let people try them.

# John Morgan

**MS:** My first question is how do you select a potency?

**JM:** Actually I use two methods. One is the intensity of the problem and also what I call the centre of gravity of it, i.e. what level it is mainly centred, physical, mental, emotional etc. For people who are on allopathic medication, I always use 30c in liquid, repeated, plussing it every day, and then I go up in threes.

**MS:** So you would give a 33c after.

**JM:** Yes. I sometimes start it with a 12c, depending on how sick they are. Also, for chronic cases with a very low vitality and a lot of pathology, then I may go solid with a 6c or 12c three times a day or twice a day. Any case where there is oversensitivity on any level then I would always go for LMs. I always start with LM1. For all other cases, if it is a mental and emotional case, I would start with 200c in split doses and then go ascending 1M, 10M, 50M, as the case develops. But I think, as I say, where there is pathology or where there is a lot of allopathic drugging, I would generally go for the liquid method.

**MS:** When you are giving remedies repeatedly, like the 30c in liquid, do you find that is OK, aggravation-wise?

**JM:** I have not had any problems with aggravation, because initially we can look at 30c and then slowly build it up.

**MS:** So do you find that if you put it into water that makes it more gentle?

**JM:** Yes, less aggravating in most cases, but I still use an LM for a very sensitive case, although there is actually no logic to that, because LMs, although they are fairly low potencies are quite strong dynamically because they have been succussed so much. They can aggravate because they are potent. They are very dynamic, although they are low in potency.

**MS:** Does your pharmaceutical background improve your understanding of how to use homeopathic potencies?

**JM:** I do not think so, to be honest. The only insight I would say is that I really consider potency to be less and less important. There are three things. Firstly I see that the potency is not that relevant to the grand scheme of things. I mean 90% is the remedy choice versus 10% the potency. Secondly, although Hahnemann talks in the *Organon* about dosage i.e. the quantity that they get, I have not seen any significant validation of what his observations are, i.e. ten granules is more aggravating than one. But I have definitely seen the weakening effect: that potencies will be less aggravating when you put them in liquid.

**MS:** Don't they become more powerful if they are diluted further?

**JM:** Well no, because the initial dilution without succussion is weakening. The number of molecules that touch the nerves of the mouth is less, because you are spreading it out over a bigger body of liquid. The whole of the LM philosophy was sub-dividing that little granule into divided doses, but of course when you start the succussion process then there is an intensifying, a dynamising, of the potency which of course raises it because you have done quite a big dilution in the beginning. So I can certainly verify that. I can also verify an LM in granules given dry on the tongue is very potent and very aggravating. Not gentle. I did some experiments on some very robust cases and got some quite strong reactions which were out of proportion to what they should have been.

I use a lot of mother tinctures and I have had more physical aggravations with mother tinctures than higher potencies. This is because people can have a material sensitivity too. It is more a sort of digestive upset or more of a toxic reaction rather than a healing aggravation. Certainly lower potencies can be quite aggravating.

**MS:** Have you come to any other conclusions about potency or dosage?

**JM:** I've observed physical antidoting factors, i.e. sunlight, heat, X-rays etc ... They validate the memory of water and also confirm that there is a saturation point. I got this through using LMs, that after ten days, or sometimes a fortnight, it is very common that the improvement plateaus, slows down a bit and then it kicks in again when you go to the next level, which infers that after about one hundred succussions of the stock bottle there is a saturation; there is a finite amount of development of the potency that liquids hold. But in contrast when you are grinding in a mortar, the trituration will go much further. With a solid you have got a much bigger surface area that keeps developing as you grind. You have got more dense molecules on the lactose where potency is and the identity of the remedy is stored. By contrast, in liquid the molecules are less dense and you have only a finite number of water and alcohol molecules that can have the capacity of developing potency.

So I think there is definitely a threshold with liquid but not so much with solids, and that is why Hahnemann moved to the trituration. Also these recent experiments where Alize Timmerman and people have been going to the C4 trituration. They have had much more dynamic results from the remedy when they have triturated the C4 and then put it into liquid, because the trituration does dynamise much, much more. It is a better medium for dynamising.

**MS:** If you have given a remedy and it has not worked, do you ever change the potency rather than the remedy?

**JM:** When you say it hasn't worked, that is very rare. My criterion for changing a remedy is if there are new symptoms they have never had before. I find that is a really good guide. If new symptoms come up that they have never had before, even if they are from the remedy - maybe it could be a proving symptom - then I would change the remedy. If nothing happened I would go quite a bit longer before I am convinced and use the new symptom as the guide.   Or of course a declining relapse. If there is relapsing and the chronic is just going on and on, if it is not turning round. I think the answer to the question is, No I won't. Occasionally I will give the next potency along but I tend to keep them going on what they are on for a bit longer until I am absolutely sure.

**MS:** Are you more likely to change the remedy rather than the potency if you are not getting satisfactory results?

**JM:** Yes, I guess so. Which I think is a common weakness actually. I think quite often the remedies change too quickly as a generalisation.

**MS:** Have you ever had aggravations where symptoms have intensified post the remedy but it hasn't gone on to be curative, nothing has sort of developed from that point.

**JM:** Well, I don't consider that an aggravation then. In sensitives, yes definitely. I've seen two very memorable patients who are very sensitive and proved all the remedies and certainly had a dose and then were ill basically.

**MS:** And then what did you do?

**JM:** Well I continued to try and turn it round with sniffing LMs with very very small doses.

**MS:** And did you achieve what you needed to achieve?

**JM:** To a degree. Using sensitive remedies which have a reputation, like *Nitric acid*, particularly has a good reputation for over-sensitive cases, but sniffing the LM from the glass was very successful in one case.

**MS:** And previous to that you were giving a centesimal and then you got them to sniff an LM?

**JM:** Yes.

**MS:** As we are talking about sensitive people, do you have any ways of identifying a sensitive case before you prescribe for them?

**JM:** Well usually there are a few clues, but not always. I mean obviously sensitivity to food and environment is a good clue, the ME, candida type generally tend to be sensitive to remedies, so that is an obvious clue, but of course there is the psychic and emotional sensitivity.

**MS:** You talked to me a little bit about dosage. Is there anything else you can tell me about how often you use and repeat remedies?

**JM:** Well, when people are on something that is repeating, if it is a chronic case, or if it is a liquid remedy, it doesn't matter how often they repeat, as long as there is some succussion before every dose. I do say with a liquid remedy they can repeat as and when they want. They can be very flexible and if they feel they don't want to have a dose today or they want to have an extra dose I give them the freedom to do that. It is fairly rare that I give solid remedies repeated, but when I do I usually tell them to stop if there is any aggravation or any new symptoms in a similar way that you would with giving liquids. So, I just see repetition in either solid or liquid as the same principle really, in terms of assessing when they stop or change.

**MS:** When you repeat a curative remedy what makes you change the potency?

**JM:** Well, what happens is they slow down, the improvement plateaus. You can see it very clearly, often there has been a period of amelioration and then there has been some change and then it slows down. Then I consider that their susceptibility has been fully satisfied and they are ready for the next step.

**MS:** Do you always go up in potency?

**JM:** Yes.

**MS:** Always?

**JM:** Again I know descending potencies is how Hahnemann used it. It is a useful method but I haven't used it to be honest.

**MS:** My final question is, do you have any questions on potency and dosage that you would like answered?

**JM:** I would like to know how the graduation of potency develops in the sense of the difference between a 200c and a 30c. In terms of its degree of refinement, in terms of its nature. I would like to know what potency is. I would like to know what its nature is. I would love it to be measured.

**MS:** Do you know why we use 30c, 200c, 1M, 10M?

**JM:** I think it was purely Kent's choice. He also used 1Ms and 5Ms and sometimes 2Ms. According to Julian Winston, who is a homeopathic historian, it is simply because that is where they stopped the machine.

# Mike Bridger

**MS:** My first question is how do you select a potency, which method do you favour?

**MB:** I don't have a method as such. I just do what is appropriate. So it would depend on what I was treating, on loads of considerations. I suppose I stick to the Kentian, Hahnemannian type thing. I don't use descending doses or anything like that.

**MS:** So when you say Kentian, Hahnemannian, you mean the more mental/emotional the case is, the higher the potency?

**MB:** Not necessarily. I mean that would be true if there wasn't any pathology and so on and I had got very clear mental symptoms, but I would say the clearer the indication for the remedy, the higher I'm prepared to go, unless I was concerned about aggravations.

**MS:** In what situation would you be concerned about an aggravation?

**MB:** Pathology, underlying pathology. Very sensitive patients. A kind of toxic feel to the case. Already on allopathic medication controlling things like asthma.  So then I would tend to keep it lower.

**MS:**   Lower and repeated or just one-off doses?

**MB:**   It depends again on the case, to some extent, but the lower I go, the more I'd be prepared to repeat. But that repetition would relate to the speed of the disease process as far as I am concerned. That would be one consideration, if something was moving quite quickly then I would repeat more quickly.

**MS:**   Like in an acute?

**MB:**   Yes.

**MS:**   Does your choice of potency ever let you down?

**MB:**   I have to say hardly ever.   As far as I'm concerned, I don't think it is the main thing.  I think if a potency doesn't work then it is the remedy rather than the potency.

**MS:**   So in situations where you have given a remedy in a particular potency and it has not worked you will change the remedy and not the potency?

**MB:**   Yes.

**MS:**   Have you ever had any situations where you have changed the potency and you have got a remedy to work in that way?

**MB:**   I might have had once or twice in about twenty years.

**MS:**   Would you ever prescribe a high potency for a sensitive patient?

**MB:**   Well, I would say in an over-sensitive patient you would be mad to go higher. It would depend on what the sensitivity is. I mean if it is a reasonably healthy sensitivity, and if they are throwing out characteristic symptoms,  then you can go high, but in an over-sensitive patient, Hahnemann is really clear to stay low.

**MS:**   When you have a patient who aggravates do you ever prescribe for that patient or will you uniformly wait?

**MB:**   Again, it is always down to the patient, isn't it?  It depends. I would try and give it as much time as the patient felt they could give it within reason, but I would not hesitate to prescribe on it if I felt it appropriate.  Very often if it is an aggravation and it isn't

161

going to sort itself out, it will produce symptoms of another remedy.

**MS:** Do you ever give a lower potency?

**MB:** I did in the early days but it was never very successful for me to be honest.

**MS:** Have you every gone up in potency?

**MB:** Yes, I will do that.

**MS:** Can you tell me what circumstances you will tend to do that in?

**MB:** Yes, in fact it just happened quite recently. Where the person has gone in too cautiously, with a low potency and it started to kick off the case but it either wasn't repeated enough or it wasn't high enough to take the case through to improvement. So, in an over-cautious situation, you can do well to go higher. If the symptoms still match the remedy and there is a clear aggravation without amelioration, and you know that is not to do with a miasm or maintaining cause or anything like that, then I think it is a really good idea to go high. Particularly in things like eczema where people tend to be very frightened of it and they go in with 30c or something. Then the case starts to aggravate, they don't repeat it, they panic, when actually they should just go in with a 1M and that will usually take it right through.

**MS:** What are your views on dosage?

**MB:** You have to keep an open mind, let the patient define those sort of things. Again it depends on the case. I obviously prefer to give a split dose or a single dose to start off with if I have got a reasonably healthy patient, and it doesn't look like there are going to be too many problems. So, if you have got a good patient and you have got a good prognosis, I do that. But as we know it is hardly ever like that, so I could repeat. I might repeat weekly. I might use more than one remedy in some cases. You know it varies very much with the patient.

**MS:** So what would make you want to repeat it more often?

**MB:** Very high energy. Often with kids. Hyperactivity. On allopathic medication. With people where I have used a low potency, I would repeat much more often, especially where there is pathology to shift.

**MS:**  Do you ever repeat high potencies often?

**MB:**  In fast moving situations like acutes and again with those very high Tubercular - type kiddies, yes.

**MS:**  Do you ever use LMs and plussing remedies and water remedies, that sort of thing?

**MB:**  I haven't done the plussing but I use LMs sometimes.

**MS:**  In your opinion what is an indication for an LM?

**MB:**  I don't actually feel it is all that much different from using a low potency like 6c or something repeated, but I think I tend to use it where there is need for great caution and the possibility of an aggravation.

**MS:**  Repeated?

**MB:**  Yes.

**MS:**  Coming back to sensitive people, apart from the obvious, which is somebody coming in and saying that whatever they take they always react very strongly to, do you have any other ways of identifying them before you treat them?

**MB:**  Well, the remedies around the case would be a bit of an indication. The patients' reactions to everything. You often find lots of  modalities, lots of reactions to lots of things, whether it is food or weather, those kind of things will indicate a very sensitive case.

**MS:**  You mentioned you sometimes use more than one remedy, when are you likely to do that?

**MB:**  Sometimes I will find things like a *Phosphorus* case and there are also symptoms of *Zincum* or *Ferrum* or *Calcarea* or something like that, I might use those on a nutrional level, low potency. Almost nutritionally, like tissue salts.  On a nutritional brick laying type level, and then give indicated remedies.  Or nosodes I might repeat also, in a case where there's a clear miasm going on, and where you have got an indication for what I call the 'constitutional'.

**MS:** So I would understand *Ferrum* because there would be anaemia?

**MB:** Yes, something like that. I use *Kali phosphoricum* a lot in MS cases, whatever the indicating remedies are I'd give *Kali phosphoricum* very low as a tissue salt.

**MS:** Thank you for that. I'd like to ask you a subtle question about energy and potency. It reflects something I am trying to articulate at present. My understanding is that vitality and intense symptoms are not the same thing and that you can have a very sick person with the energy to exhibit very vivid symptoms, like a psychotic for example. At college, we were taught that energy equals high potency, but in those situations it is not quite true. Do you have an explanation?

**MB:** Well, I think although you might have intensity, and although the symptoms can be striking, actually very often what you have got is common symptoms. Particularly in mental circumstances where there are so many very strong symptoms, very strong delusions, but you will usually find that they are transient and they will change very quickly, particularly with other striking symptoms. Actually, all you can take is something like insanity or a rubric like that, because there is very little pattern to it. There is very little consistency so that the individual symptoms have become unreliable. They are nothing more than common symptoms.

**MS:** Isn't that the same sort of thing as a heart attack, lots of drama, with very visible symptoms that you could describe as energy?

**MB:** What is it? I suppose it is energy, but you are still having to find the differentiating symptoms. The intensity relates to the heart attack symptoms and so they are really quite common. What is more difficult is to find the other little symptoms round the prism that signify the remedy.

**MS:** So what you are saying is, that if the characteristic symptoms are not there, then no matter what the intensity is, prescribe low?

**MB:** Yes, you have to start prescribing therapeutically really.

**MS:** Is there anything that you would like to know about potency or dosage?

**MB:** I think there is all sorts of information coming on the market which I don't know quite why they are saying what they are saying, or where their information comes from.  It is unsubstantiated. What is written in the old authorities is absolutely fine as far as I can see. I have never found any problem with it. I think potency is secondary to getting the remedy. It is fine-tuning really.

# Robin Logan

**MS:** My first question is how do you select the potency?

**RL:** It's fairly simple, but at the same time I have to think about it, because it's such an instinctive thing now. One of my main criteria for selecting a potency is what I consider to be the potential for aggravation. So, if I consider there is potential for aggravation, for example, a skin condition that's been suppressed a lot, then I'll use a low potency. One of my favourite ones is a 12c, I use that quite a lot.

**MS:** And what dosage might you use?

**RL:** I'll give it for at least a month, perhaps twice a day for four or five weeks. I give instructions to contact me if things are going strange in any way.

**MS:** How often does that happen?

**RL:** Very rarely, actually, but I tend to only give repeated doses of a remedy if I feel pretty confident about the remedy selection, because I don't like the idea of giving a completely inappropriate remedy over long periods of time like that.

**MS:** And if you're not so confident of the remedy choice?

**RL:** If I'm not so confident, and if I still feel that a low potency is the most appropriate thing, I'll still give the prescription but I'll give much more advice about contacting me if they're not happy with the way things are going. Another thing that I'll do is to use 30c. I'm happier about giving a 30c once a week than giving a 12c every day, if it's the wrong remedy. Some people might say there's no difference; that giving them the wrong remedy is still giving them the wrong remedy however many times you repeat it, but I just feel happier about doing it that way.

**MS:** That's probably because your experiences have dictated that?

**RL:** Everything I do is moulded by past experience. A lot of what I do is instinctive and unconscious. I have to think quite hard about reasons for doing it. If I'm treating an every day case, where it's just a functional problem with emotional problems, I usually start with a 200c. That's my most commonly prescribed potency, because I feel that if it's the right remedy you'll get a response pretty quickly and at the same time it leaves room for going up the scale if necessary. If I could only have one potency in my whole remedy kit, that would be it.

**MS:** Have you drawn any conclusions to potencies that haven't been documented before. Do you have any of your own discoveries?

**RL:** Not really my own, but what I think I've confirmed - something that Dr. Eizayaga taught me quite a long time ago - is that you don't have to be frightened of repeating the dose. In fact if you're on the right remedy, if you give one dose of a 50M or thirty consecutive doses of a 50M, in other words once a day for a month, you're likely to get a very similar outcome, and that's something which I've experimented with and found to be the case. I don't give a remedy every day because there's no need. It's just of waste of pills and a waste of time. If one dose works, why give thirty? Not many people have actually tried doing it, but my experience concurs with Eizayaga, in that there's no reason to give a placebo if you want to give someone something to take every day and you're on the right remedy. But taking it every day won't necessarily speed things up or work any more effectively either, but neither will it do anything to spoil the treatment.

**MS:** I've had experiences where I've asked my patient to take a remedy daily for three days, and they've said that they felt OK on the first and second day, but on the third day, they started to aggravate.

**RL:** Yes, but I think that can happen even if you give a single dose. I don't think that was necessarily because you gave one too many. I've a lot less fear of over prescribing nowadays.

**MS:** What do you tend to do if a patient aggravates?

**RL:** I think it's best to do nothing if possible, and just let things run their course. If somebody really feels like they need to be doing something, my next best option would be to give a lower potency of the same remedy. So you know if someone's had a 200c or 1M or something, and they're having an aggravation and they feel like they want to do something to improve the situation, I'll tell them to go out and get a 6c from a chemist and take that for a few days. I'm not really sure what effect that has quite honestly, because it's very difficult to know what would have happened if they'd taken nothing or a placebo. But that's what I'll do if people aren't happy with just waiting.

**MS:** At the very least, you might be simply pacifying the patient?

**RL:** Yes, well that's my belief, but it's very hard to know without checking it across a really large sample of patients and comparing it to similar ones who took something else.

**MS:** If a remedy that you've prescribed doesn't work, have you ever changed the potency successfully rather than changed the remedy?

**RL:** No, I don't personally believe that that's going to make much difference. I think that it is definitely the most important thing to find the right remedy, and the right remedy will do something in any potency. The only time the correct remedy seems not to do anything in my experience is when they haven't taken enough of it. So if they're taking a low potency and then after ten days or two weeks they're saying that nothing much has changed, that's a big mistake, because a low potency can start kicking in after a month or even more, in some cases. That's why I like the 200c because I have a lot of faith that if it's the right remedy you'll see some sort of response fairly quickly, whereas if you give one dose of a 30c, I feel you could miss the effect of it. I can't remember the last time I thought a non-reaction must just be that I gave the wrong potency. I tend to assume it's the wrong remedy if nothing's happening.

**MS:**  How long do you normally wait to get a reaction then?

**RL:**  I like to wait a month. Of course it depends on the case. There are some cases where you need a quicker response than that, but in the average case I don't like to change things in less than three weeks or four weeks.

**MS:**  I've had one case, where after a month they were meant to come back and see me and they went on holiday. So they delayed the appointment for a couple of weeks, and when they came back (it was an eczema case in a child), the eczema had completely cleared up. But the remedy hadn't kicked in until they'd gone on holiday. Now originally I thought maybe it's the sun or the sea or whatever, but actually I'm still in contact with the patient, and it's never come back.

**RL:**  Patience is definitely required and I'm sure I've been guilty of being impatient in the past. There are definitely cases where you think nothing's happening and then four or five weeks on it all starts clearing up.

**MS:**  What makes you change the potency?

**RL:**  Only when things have reached a plateau. I do think that changing the potency prematurely can upset things, maybe only temporarily, but I think that is one of the mistakes you can make. I like a remedy to have completely run out of steam before I go up. On the other hand I'm not averse to repeating the same potency quite frequently. I don't necessarily wait for a complete relapse before I repeat the same potency.

**MS:**  When you say upset the case, what do you mean?

**RL:**  A relapse where symptoms start coming back or the improvement stops or something goes wrong and then it can take time for everything to settle down again. It often necessitates going back to the original potency. It's like things are coasting along at a certain rate and then you just push too hard and then everything goes off the rails.

**MS:**  And then you said you won't wait for a complete relapse to perhaps repeat the same potency, so what would be your indication for repeating a potency?

**RL:**  I'm still experimenting quite a lot with that. One thing I do a lot these days is to give a 200c every week in a case where I feel there might be either antidotal factors or just a very stuck case that I feel needs a lot of pushing and coaxing. I might repeat 200cs weekly without waiting to see what effect the first dose had. I'm still unsure about the wisdom of this. I always lean towards single doses, because if that works, it works very, very well. But it's born out of frustration, not enough people getting better quickly enough, you're always looking for ways of speeding things up and making things work better. That's one of the things I do, I repeat the same potency on a regular basis. But I suspect that's often motivated by my failing to find the right remedy more than anything else.

**MS:**   But having done that for a little while now, is it effective? Are you happy with what you're doing?

**RL:**   I'm not too sure. I still feel a bit unsure about it.

**MS:**   One of the things that I found when I was in practice early on was that remedies ran out of steam very quickly because I wasn't giving a good enough remedy. That experience made me experiment with LMs. Do you ever use LMs?

**RL:**   I have experimented with them but found them a little bit fiddly to use. I feel I have a good grasp of the centesimal scale and I know how to use it. I know when to change potency. I know which potency to go to next. I know how long roughly to expect a particular potency to work for. But I'm still in the dark with LMs and because of that I've given up using them. On the one hand people say you only ever need to give LM1 and you don't need anything else and yet, you can give LM50. I just don't understand the scale well enough to feel comfortable using it. I've found the centesimal scale has served me well, so I don't feel like I need the LMs.

**MS:**   What about plussing remedies?

**RL:**   I do that sometimes through being influenced by other people. I have experimented with that in cancer cases. The results are inconclusive.

**MS:**   What about sensitive people?

**RL:**   I've had so few of them that I haven't had the opportunity to experiment much, but my tendency has been, like most people, to give a low potency. Yes, fewer doses of low potencies because of the potential for aggravation. But the thing is I've only had a handful of those, they're nightmare patients. I don't think I've ever significantly helped any of them, because they just don't stick with it. Whatever you give them makes them worse.

**MS:** Have you ever had a situation where you've given a lower potency and even though the patient is getting better they may have a symptom that simply doesn't shift until you've given a higher potency?

**RL:** Yes, that happens all the time. You expect that when you're using lower potencies that there are certain things that will only shift once you get further up the scale.

**MS:** Something I'm trying to understand at the moment is the definition of energy. Certainly, before I started to think about this book, I equated energy with intensity. So, if somebody comes in and everything is quite vivid then to me that would be an indication of energy. It probably is, but certainly with people who are for instance, psychotic, that intensity is there and yet they are very ill. My feeling is that perhaps one shouldn't prescribe high for those types of cases. And the same perhaps if somebody is having a heart attack you might find it very dramatic and vivid, but it's not like a child with an acute. I just wondered if you have any thoughts on that?

**RL:** I wouldn't use low potencies in those cases. I use the 200c potency a lot. My feeling is that they use up remedies quickly. I saw someone yesterday with terrible sleeplessness. She's had sleep problems for thirty years and she doesn't take sleeping pills, she just doesn't go to sleep. She's a very, very hyper person, an absolute live wire who just can't sit still for a minute and her mind just doesn't shut off at night. So I gave her a 200c of *Coffea* to take at night for one month. Where there's very intense symptoms like that in an intense energetic kind of person, I will use a highish potency and repeat it very frequently.

**MS:** My very last question is do you have any questions that you would like answered about potency or dosage?

**RL:** I don't think it's the easiest question to answer - probably in fifty or one hundred years time we'll be able to answer it more easily - but I'd like to know about the different effects of potencies that are close to each other on the centesimal scale. What I mean is whether a 9c behaves differently to a 6c and a 12c and a 15c and an 18c, because there are some theories that some potencies are more calming and others more stimulating, more effective in different ways. When Benveniste was doing some of his experiments on the memory of water I think they found that there was a difference in the way that different dilutions were behaving. That would be interesting to know one day, whether there are any particular differences between these potencies, other than one just being a little bit higher and more potent than the other.

# Ian Watson

**MS:** How do you select a potency, what method do you favour?

**IW:** I would favour using a combination of factors in each case, rather than use a certain method, and that would include, for example: the age of the patient, my perception of the strength of the constitution, the depth of the pathology, any features like ongoing medication, or anything else that might interfere with the treatment. All of these factors are what I would look at, but the main thing for me would be the clarity of the prescribing image.

**MS:** The age of the patient would be, the younger the patient the higher the potency?

**IW:** In general, yes, but that could be overridden, for example by constitutional strength. If I saw an older person but they had good vitality and they weren't on drugs and the picture was clear, I would give them a high potency too.

**MS:** Can you clarify the perception of the constitution?

**IW:** My in-the-moment, snapshot-understanding of what that person's underlying constitutional strength is. Obviously I am making a best guess at that, because in reality you don't know what that is until you've started treating the person.

**MS:** So are we talking about the vital force, the strength of the vital force? The energy there or...?

**IW:** Yes, I guess you could put it that way. I tend to just talk about constitutional strength and I don't really use the term vital force that much, because it's relatively immeasurable isn't it?

**MS:** When you talk about the constitutional strength, do you mean certain types of constitution, certain remedy pictures...?

**MS:** No, it's irrespective of remedy picture. I am talking about the *underlying strength of the body itself*. So, I have an assumption there that some bodies are built better than others and my experience supports that. Is it someone who is very sensitive and relatively fragile, or is it someone who is basically robust? That is what I am looking at. It is has nothing to do with the remedy picture.

**MS:** Right, to clarify, if you have someone who is relatively robust they would get...?

**IW:** They are more likely to get a higher potency, unless there are other factors that over-rule that. For example, they are taking loads of drugs or something similar.

**MS:** And sensitivity would go the other way, would it?

**IW:** Exactly.

**MS:** Depth of pathology is an interesting one and something I am trying to get my head around at the moment. Are you familiar with Dr Ramakrishnan's book on cancer?

**IW:** I know of its existence but I have not read it.

**MS:** He tends to use 200c potency plussed and repeated for cancer, and that is a highish potency and a deep pathology. He is getting very good results, so I am still learning around that area. Do you have any sort of information that you can share about pathology and potency with me?

**IW:** For me, its an open question because I studied the book *Principles of Prescribing* by Mathur. I studied that years ago and it gives examples of different prescribers, one of whom was a high potency prescriber, I think he was an Indian, and he was treating mostly advanced pathologies using 50Ms and CMs. I was exposed to that early on in my homeopathic career, and I always had this thought in the back of my mind, well why not? The results seem to be suggesting that that is quite do able.

Then again, I have also studied with Eizayaga, who would say that in serious pathologies you want to start with a 3c and 6c and you can always work your way up. So for me, I think that depth of pathology is a factor, but not necessarily an overriding one. I would say that even in a case of advanced pathology, if the picture is clear and there are no other interfering factors like being overdosed with chemotherapy or something of that kind, then I would not necessarily go against using high potencies. Similarly, if there is a lot of pain or intensity in the situation I am more likely to use high potencies, because in my experience the body will burn it up quickly in that instance. The only time I would really favour the low potencies exclusively would be if I think the person needs a lot of doses on a regular basis, and that's usually because they are on a lot of medication.

**MS:** What about aggravations then, especially if you are using very high potencies?

**IW:** I don't think aggravation is a function of potency primarily. I mean, some of the most difficult to handle aggravations I have experienced have been with clients who have been on 30c. Sometimes lower than that. You know, I have had people take one dose of a 6c and all hell breaks out, so you can't say that its just from high potencies. Some of the most gentle cures I've seen have been from 1Ms and 10Ms, and sometimes even 200cs, and with no aggravation whatsoever.

So I've let go of the idea that high potencies aggravate and low potencies don't. I think that is more determined by things like the sensitivity of the patient, and also the expectation of the prescriber. I think that's a big factor. You know sometimes we set people up to aggravate, so they do. I have had people aggravate on Sac lac, just to kind of prove to myself that that was possible. I have actually experimented with that, sometimes with patients who are highly suggestible and also sensitive types, and they will aggravate on anything. So I think potency is a secondary thing as far as aggravation goes.

**MS:** Sensitivity is a big issue, isn't it, for us homeopaths. Have you got any information to share with us on that?

**IW:** Sensitivity to me is the same as susceptibility. It's another way of looking at that phenomenon. So, on the one hand it's the bane of our lives because we are always wondering, is this a sensitive patient or not? But at the same time, we need a degree of sensitivity otherwise we don't get any response at all. So understanding a person's type of sensitivity I think is one of the most crucial things about case taking. To me that is more important than gathering a list of symptoms. It's getting a sense of, not only *how* sensitive they are, but what is the *nature* of their sensitivity. In other words what are they sensitive to, what is it that makes them a unique individual?

**MS:** And I guess it's this sensitivity that leads you to the remedy.

**IW:** Absolutely, it's one of the key things that will formulate the remedy picture. For example, if you have a list of food sensitivities we associate that with a certain remedy type, but I also look at in a more general sense. Some people are more sensitive to the weather, some people are sensitive to the presence of the homeopath, some are not.

**MS:** I believe you have to be very, very clear about what you want to give really sensitive people otherwise they are going to aggravate, but if you get the remedy right, and the potency and dosage right, then I don't think they will. What do you think?

**IW:** That is an interesting belief. I have really studied this a lot with different practitioners, and I tend to find that our patients confirm the unconsciously-held beliefs of the practitioners to a large extent. So if you believe that 'if I get the remedy right, they won't aggravate', that will be your experience. Whereas I know other homeopaths who believe that if you get the remedy slightly wrong, that will create a big aggravation, so they have a different belief which their practice experience will tend to confirm. So to me it is worth uncovering what kind of assumption you hold about what you think will happen, because you will tend to see that mirrored in your practice. I know from my own experience that when I change my internal reality around it, then what happens to the people I am treating changes too.

**MS:** I suppose my internal reality should therefore be that all my patients are going to get better and not aggravate?

**IW:** You could choose that one. I came around to the realisation that some people will, it seems, as part of their healing process, need to aggravate. And in that sense, this is something which is independent of us even though we influence it. I know that some people feel they haven't got their money's worth if they don't aggravate. In the north of England, it's quite popular for people to think they need to suffer a bit in order to feel well, and I don't want to take that away from them. So the kind of strategy that I tend to adopt is that people will get well in whatever way is right for them, rather than me saying that they should never aggravate or they should always aggravate. And the ones that do aggravate - if you let it be OK, then it generally is. It's not really about whether they aggravate or not – it's whether you and they are OK with the fact that they aggravate.

**MS:** I think that is true and I think as you become more experienced as a homeopath that is easier to do.

**IW:** Yes, you become less worried about those things and you tend to think, 'Oh yeah, it's just an aggravation, it's fine, it will pass', rather than losing sleep over it.

**MS:** What do you actually do with aggravations, do you always wait or do ...?

**IW:** No, I don't always do anything. I think if you always do something then you are an allopath not a homeopath. For me homeopathy is about individualising everything, so there is no always and there is no never.

**MS:** In that case what would make you wait if somebody aggravates?

**IW:** If the person is doing fine. If they are OK with the fact that they are aggravating, then it's none of my business and I tend to work that way. I don't make myself particularly available. People know that ahead of time and they have to be fairly self-responsible in order to work with me in the first place. Which means, if something comes up and I am not around, then they must be willing to ride it, or to deal with it in their own way. If they get a lot of pain or something and they can't handle it, then they know it is OK with me for them to take painkillers if they need to, or they can prescribe a first aid remedy if they need that for themselves. I don't make it that conditional that they have to wait for instructions from me. I tend to trust that people will do what they need to do, and I will support them in whatever that is.

**MS:** What about somebody who actually finds you who has an aggravation and they don't want to put up with it?

**IW:** I prescribe on it.

**MS** Do you change the remedy?

**IW:** I tend to just look at the image that's being thrown up, because I find that a lot of what people call 'aggravation' is actually just another state that they have gone into. So it's not an aggravation at all but is in fact another layer that has been thrown up. Therefore, I tend to act as though I don't know what remedy they have taken before, and say to myself, If I had never seen this person before in my life, what would I give them now? And I give them that. So if it's midnight and they are freaking out, I give them *Arsenicum album* or *Aconite*, regardless of the fact that they may have been given *Calcarea Carbonica* six hours ago. I find this works pretty well, and you can prescribe without prejudice.

**MS:** If a remedy does not work at all, have you ever stuck with that remedy because you felt it's still indicated or the best for them, and changed the potency?

**IW:** Yes, although I would say that is pretty rare. Usually if a person says that it hasn't worked at all, obviously sometimes we find out that in fact it has, but they just didn't notice. If it has really not done anything, usually I find that means that they have not been given enough of it, if I am sure it's the right thing. So, if I have started with a low potency - say they are taking a 6c and they have only had one or two doses - well it's reasonable that it hasn't done anything yet, so they maybe just need to take more. But if they have taken a reasonably high potency and it hasn't done anything and they have waited what to me is a reasonable time (and I don't have any fixed criteria of that, a reasonable amount of time in one case might be a day and in another case it might be a couple of weeks), then I am more inclined to change the remedy. I am not asking the patient to wait around for months.

**MS;** I don't think most patients are either.

**IW:** Neither do I. They pay good money to have something happen and if absolutely nothing has happened I tend not to stick with it. I tend to say, well OK, I have missed something here.

**MS:** What are your views on dosage?

**IW:** You mean repetition?

**MS:** Yes.

**IW:** I think it's a guessing game when you start out, and to me the best approach is that you just start with your best guess but you give the patient permission to modify it themselves. That's the way I found works best for me, and for the patient. It is much better than me being in charge of it, pretending that I know what is best! I just say, we'll start on this basis, you know, once a day, three times a day, once a week, whatever it is, but as soon as you feel like something is moving I want you to monitor it yourself. If you feel like you are taking too much, you cut it down. If you feel like it is not doing much you can increase it. I build that in right from the beginning. Then they report back to me with what they found was their optimum dosage.

**MS:** So, if you are starting off with higher potencies, but not very high potencies, say 30cs and 200cs for example, would you tend to give one-off or repeat in that situation? How would you start?

**IW:** I would make a guess as to how much I thought they would need in order to get the ball rolling. So, if all the factors are favourable - they have good constitutional strength, a clear remedy picture, nothing in the way, no drugs - then I may well give a single dose and this should be enough in this case to at least see where it is going. Where the underlying vitality is weak, the remedy picture is a bit hazy, they are taking medication or have been, things of that kind, I am more than likely to give it repeated for a few days until they feel it working. Here it is more the idea of kick-starting the constitution, because it is likely they will need it. If my guess is that they are going to be a bit sluggish, then I say start to take it two, three or four times a day for a few days, and I will give them enough doses for three, four, five days. I tell them, once you feel the treatment is on the way, then you can stop. So I will leave it up to them.

**MS:** If someone is on medication I normally give an LM, but if someone is on medication and you are giving a 30c for example and you kick-started it, do you find the medication can interfere with it later on and the remedy has a very short life span, or not necessarily?

**IW:** No, I don't think it's the remedy life span. I don't think remedies *have* a life span! To me that is a bit of a myth. I think that individual people have varying degrees of ability to respond, and that's both to remedies and to other substances like drugs and so on. Some people, even though they are on medication, will take a remedy and sail through it, whereas for someone else, the fact that they are on medication will slow everything down for them. To me it's not that the drug is interfering with the remedy, but that it's affecting their system on a daily basis. If you only give the remedy once, and every day following they are taking something that is powerfully impinging on their system, the chances are they are going to need more of that remedy in order to keep improving. You know, it's like a counter balance. I don't believe that these substances interfere with our remedies. There is nothing there for them to interfere with.

**MS:** When you repeat a remedy, what makes you want to change the potency?

**IW:** They have had enough of it. They have done well up to a point and they seem to plateau or they start to slip back, and the remedy picture has not altered substantially, so they still need the same remedy. What they are saying is that they have had enough of it at that level. And I don't pretend to know in advance whether that will happen, or when it will happen.

**MS:** Just wait for the patient to tell you really.

**IW:** I give them permission to detect that and to let me know, because all the times I changed it on my own accord, it's usually been premature and I've regretted it. So, I have learnt to keep my hands off. If they want to take a 6c for six months and do well on it, then that's fine with me now.

**MS:** Do you ever use water-potencies? Do you use LMs or plus remedies?

**MS:** I have done. I found that these are things that I do in a phase and then I suppose I get bored with it and I go back to giving pills. I have experimented quite a bit, more so with centesimals in liquid form and less so with things like LMs, although I have used LMs as well.

**MS:** After experimenting, what would make you want to give a water-potency now?

**IW:** If I haven't got many pills left, I wouldn't want to give the whole bottle away! That's the main one. The other would be over-sensitivity of the client, for example, someone who describes themselves as the type who will over-respond to anything in a normal dose. That to me is a way of diluting it a little bit further, and it gives them more adjustment possibilities. They can vary the amount of drops if they have got a dropper bottle. So I use it for people who seem to need that fine-tuning, but I would say that it's not that common.

**MS:** Do you find that it makes the remedy more gentle if you put it in water?

**IW:** It does when it does. It doesn't always.

**MS:**   Do you have any questions on dosage or on potency that you would like answered?

**IW:**   Yes, there was some interesting work that came out a couple of years ago where Tony Pinkus from Ainsworths was involved in some research and there was a suggestion that potency did not go up in a linear scale, which is what we have been taught. You know, the idea that it starts at the tincture and it goes up to infinity via 6c, 30c and 200c etc. Rather than it being linear in that sense, it had more of the shape of a kind of wave form, with peaks and troughs. That was something that intrigued me, but I would still have an open mind about it. The suggestion being that a 200c, for example, could in fact be 'higher' than a 1M. Which was interesting to me because there is a lot of folklore in homeopathy that says that 200c is the one that really aggravates and that 1Ms are relatively gentle, and my own limited experience would go along with that to some extent.

So that would be an open question for me that I'd be interested to have answered. Whether in fact potency isn't this linear thing, and that 'higher' doesn't necessarily mean 'higher'. And I don't know what the answer is or whether there is any research that has drawn any good conclusions about that. But I remember it raising a question in my mind that intrigued me. It would be worth knowing, wouldn't it? And it might give some explanation as to why some of these high potency prescribers can give what we would classify as very high potencies with great frequency and apparently no problems. You know, maybe they are not as high as we think.

**MS:**   To be honest with you when I look through all my old cases, I tend to have more aggravation in the lower potencies, or the medium potencies.

**IW:**   That has been my experience – interesting, huh?

**MS:**   But then could that be because I am normally really sure of my remedy when I give a high potency?

# Francis Treuherz

**MS:**     What is your method for choosing a potency?

**FT:**     A frequent method, but not the best method, is drawer homeopathy. The potency that happens to be in the drawer when the patient is here. Sometimes a patient needs a remedy urgently because something is happening acutely, so you just use what is in the drawer and it often works, which seems to demonstrate that potency is sometimes less important than the remedy. But then the factor is how frequently is the remedy going to be repeated or needed because the potency was not actually the optimum one.

Sometimes I give the wrong potency. I had a patient who came on a GP referral, for coughing blood. On taking the case, he was male and gay and HIV positive and he had chronic liver disease on which they had given up. He was indeed coughing and it was not a question of 'organ support', it was a question of selecting the correct remedy and I went through the case and decided on *Carduus marianus*, because it has pain on the left lobe of the liver which is near the centre of the abdomen, which is where his pain was, and because it has liver and lung symptoms. *Chelidonium* is the other lobe of the liver but has pain in the shoulder. So it was a careful choice. I gave him a 6c potency to take three times a day and nothing happened. I wanted a phone call from him very quickly for results. So, then I gave him mother tincture and it worked. I went to Clarke's *Materia Medica* and thought hard about what was needed in this case and I gave him mother tincture. It was a chronic illness but the prescription had to work quickly, that was drawer homeopathy gone wrong, but I did not have mother tincture; we got it from Ainsworth's, very quickly.

**MS:** So was it what Clarke said that made you go down in potency rather than up in potency?

**FT:** I probably read Burnett as well, because Clarke writes about these remedies having heard about them from Burnett. There are just a few remedies I use from time to time in mother tincture. *Crataegus* is one and Clarke says you can use it for months, although you do have to monitor, even in mother tincture. *Spartium scoparium*, gorse or broom, a prickly yellow plant, to be used for high blood pressure. Years ago, I read up a case by a GP called Dr R.A.F. Jack, whom I since got to know personally, and it is now published in his book *Homeopathy in General Practice*. But it was an old article, in the *British Homeopathic Journal*, and the person's remedy appeared to be *Sulphur*, but he was given the plant-based mother tincture (of *Spartium scoparium*) to help reduce the blood pressure and I have done that too.

I was also in India and I was in Goa, it used to be a Portuguese colony, and there was this guy in the bar on holiday and he was eating olives and there was a little dish into which he was spitting the stones, and I thought great I shall eat an olive, but it was not an olive at all. So, what was it? It was *jambol* fruit, *Syzygium jambolanum*, a remedy used in diabetes and the sweetest thing you have ever tasted. A terribly sweet little fruit, *Syzygium jambolanum* is very good for diabetes, for reducing blood sugar in someone who is on insulin, it helps stabilise. It will not necessarily always get them off insulin, it is not always curable, but that is another mother tincture I use. The mother tinctures are not all from Burnett. I cannot immediately think of another, although occasionally there will have been others that I use in mother tincture. It is not simply organ support, a theory without much weight in my opinion. It is actually using the remedies exactly from the materia medica.

I have just tidied away a book on my French shelf, called *Low Potency and Drainage in Homeopathy* (*Basses Dilutions et Drainage en Homéopathie*) and it is an attempt to understand where the idea originates. It has seven hundred footnotes, so there is the whole literature on why to give low potencies.

Obviously the substances are not toxic and they are usually plant-based. One is not going to give a mother tincture of *Arsenicum album*. Some of them are plants which may have been used homeopathically, unconsciously by herbalists, like the Indian use of *Syzygium jambolanum*, which have then had provings. Another very, very low potency remedy that I learnt about in Calcutta, although I had read about it in Boericke, is called *Ficus religiosa*, which is a fig tree. It is not an English fig, the religious bit is an Ayurvedic belief. An Indian homeopath observed a dog eating the leaves and it coughed up blood immediately. They use it in road traffic accidents in a 1x.

Somebody came through the front door of my home carrying a box of groceries and the door was made of glass and he omitted to open it first, so I gave him a *Ficus religiosa* 1x and it stopped the bleeding. He needed some stitches but they did not have to worry about the bleeding. Another remedy to consider is *Sabal serrulata* in enlarged prostate. So that is the value of the low potencies.

My potency selection uses the whole range up to very occasionally higher than 10M. The highest potencies are often used when the mental/emotional and physical symptoms overlap, but they are not always the first potencies used. If I am using high potencies I might start with a 1M to give me room to go up to the 10M and vary occasionally the 50M.

Sometimes in a very acute state I might go straight in with a high potency and I will mention a case in a moment. I often give 6c, 30c, 200c, 1M, as the first potency depending on what it is and occasionally an LM.

**MS:** Can you tell me why you do that?

**FT:** Yesterday somebody came in with psoriasis, which he had had for eight years, but only in three places, the one knee and two elbows. Two weeks previously it spread and it looked like an enormous rash of drops all over his arms and legs. There was an emotional cause. He was not particularly well educated and did not understand much about homeopathy. He was an electrician with a heart of gold, a very warm personality, but if I then change the metaphor, he was 'the salt of the earth'. I gave him *Natrum muriaticum*.

His mother had died of cancer and that had been the onset and his daughter had had her first birthday two weeks before and she had been moping around because her grandmother was not there. But I did not give him the LM, which I often do, because of what the allopaths call compliance. Not everyone is happy with going through the shaking stuff.

What I gave him was *Natrum muriaticum* 6c to be taken 3 times a day. I gave him two bottles of the 6c so that he had one at home and one in his bag; so that when he forgets he can still take one. I did this so that there would be compliance. I also told him not to worry if he still forgot to take one. He was in touch with all sorts of noxious things, clambering under furniture and plumbing to put in electric cables, so he needed a low potency regularly.

The previous day, sitting in that chair, was a patient with psoriasis, a *Natrum muriaticum,* whom I first saw ten or so years before, who had done very well on LMs. He was a quiet thoughtful A level student at the time, who was delighted with the ritual, an intellectual and reserved young man. He came back this time after a gap of some years with psoriatic arthropathy.

Apparently, the psoriasis returned. He had gone to the allopaths. He had surgery on his knee, which he regretted, and then came back to me. I put him straight on to LM 6 or 7, taking up from where he had left off and he was perfectly happy and he had said, "I do not know why I spent the fee, I could have done that myself." But he will be back. A faithful patient.

The thing about LM is chronic illness, my fear of aggravation and a knowledge or hunch that there will be compliance. I used the LMs exactly how John Morgan wrote about them in an article in *The Homeopath* that I commissioned when I was editor, only ten years ago, when he was called John Tomlinson; on *Dose, Dilution and the LM potencies (Vol. 10 No. 4. December 1990)*. Which is in 150ml of water, shake it thoroughly, with rigour, and one teaspoon of that into water, stir it and sip it each evening. When one potency is finished, you go up to the next.

I do not do funny things like starting with LM18 or whatever else people have concocted. I just stick to the book and John Morgan is one of the most experienced, as it were, on the LMs. I do not use them a lot. I do not keep them in stock, and I always order them from the pharmacy. This is partly because I formerly worked above a pharmacy in Finchley, and I used to work close to a pharmacy, Ainsworth's in Central London, so that I have not as vast a stock of remedies as some people.

**MS:**   Have you ever had anyone aggravating on an LM?

**FT:** Occasionally, and I will say to them, have a gap, wait for the aggravation to die down and try every other day, or if you feel that you can monitor yourself, take a dose, wait for reaction, and then take another when you need it. But usually, they go back to a routine like every other day.

I do not often use a 6c. I often use a 30c and a 200c, because I do not often do a 'take a remedy daily' prescription. I get a lot of people with complaints that one would think might be acutes, but they have had them for a week or two and they have tried self-help and then they come in desperation. So it is the end of a cough, then the end of a cold, or it might be the early stages of something painful like arthritis. I might start with a 30c. I shall say to take one daily for a week but I will write this underlined, <u>stop if there is a reaction</u>. I always use written prescriptions with my face to face patients. Patients receive a copy of the prescription based on an NHS prescription layout. Having worked in the NHS I have realised how important it was for patients to have a written prescription. I used to write things on a compliment slip, but I write all my instructions on this. I use it as a receipt as well.

**MS:** Even when you give the remedy you write the instructions on here as well?

**FT:** Oh yes. So they know the name of it and they know what they are taking. If they have to ring the help line or call someone it's important that they have the name of it.

So, I will write down 30c one daily for a week and stop if you get a reaction. If they are new, I will say of a reaction, "It may be a good or a bad reaction and I am not going to tell you what reaction to expect as this might provoke that type of a reaction. If you are in doubt ring me and if I am not available then call the help line." You see, part of the potency is follow-up, and that means being available seven days a week, whether it is me or my call service because that is important with new patients.

There is a way of prescribing ascending potencies and technical ways of describing a collective single split dose and so on. I never use the jargon. I do not use the language and I very rarely do the going up scale thing, because afterwards I sort of scratch my head and think, well which one was the right one? I have just given three, is the next potency going to be another 10M, because I've gone up one, two, three?

I know we were taught this at college, and occasionally one sees it in old American journals, but I prefer to give someone the same potency, and stick to it. For me the best teaching guide to potency were the Greeks. I think it was the spoken lectures originally and then the collected writings of Vasilis Ghegas. He was a colleague of George Vithoulkas. There is a strange tale to it. My uncle was the Dean of the Athens University Medical School and he taught Vasilis allopathy before he became a homeopath. There was an immediate affinity when I first met Vasilis. He was very clear, if a potency is working, stick to it. If the interval between needing repetition of doses is getting shorter, then you either need to change the remedy or the potency. You may or may not need to re-take the case.

So, if the same remedy is still needed, it is time to go up and that is what I do. I have been up to a 10M with someone who I started on a 6c and I occasionally used the 12c as well. Where the diagnosis had been epilepsy, we are of course worried about aggravations. This woman used to come with headaches and she had not had a convulsion for a long time, but often had what she thought was the pre-convulsive state. We got up to a 10M and she had been taking it rather too frequently, so I went back down to 12c, which was a Vasilis' idea. The remedy worked again. I did not even go up to 50M. So literally, maybe eight or ten times over a year and a half we had gone up to a 10M and then down again and then the 12c did the trick. So I may start with a 30c, 200c, 1M and go up gradually if the remedy is right and the potency is exhausted.

**MS:** So when you got to that 10M and you had the indication to go down to the 12c, was it that she was experiencing an aggravation?

**FT:** No, the remedy was not working. Or rather, it was working but it was not working very long. There seemed no future in taking a 10M every day and so I went back down again and then one dose held for ages. We are talking about someone who came to me as a university student and is now married with children, so it's been fifteen years since I have been seeing her. Not so often now, although she occasionally comes back for the children, but there is loads of self-help.

**MS:** So, just to get it right, the remedy was working but it just had a very, very short life span, but it was not that it was not working.

**FT:** That's right. It's like it got exhausted going up the scale, so I needed to come down again. But what I cannot remember, is which 19th century classic source that idea probably came from.

I have never used things like descending scales. Let's talk about the use of high potencies, in a severe life-threatening acute. A patient felt funny for a week, in his abdomen, and did not really know what was happening. He had tried one or two of the self help remedies. He was at a meeting where those present included medical doctors, one of them was a homeopath, and he literally collapsed. He said, I don't know what to do, will you look after me please? The doctor took one look at him and laid him out on the committee table, cleared the room, examined him and decided he was seriously ill. Not being prepared to wait for the ambulance, the doctor put him in his car and took him to St Mary's. Someone else telephoned the hospital to expect him.

It was peritonitis. The patient had the problem on the left. It was not the appendix, but it was the same sort of thing as a burst appendix. All the classic symptoms. The doctors prescribed intravenous Metronidazole, Flagyl, and surgery before the prescription was given. Obviously they wanted to take various samples, get ready for Dracula to come, the phlebotomist and so on. Anyhow, the patient permitted his blood to be taken but refused the operation. So they decided they needed two doctors to detain him against his will using mental health legislation as he was deemed a danger to himself and others.

The patient staggered out of the hospital, and went home against the advice of a medical doctor, Dr John Ball who used to teach medical sciences at the College of Homeopathy. And against the advice of *even* his homeopath, the patient took *Pyrogenium* 10M. He was at first grey and green by turns and a couple of hours later, he was merely pale. He did take the precaution of getting the Metronidazole (from a prescription) as a suppository, in case it did not work. Anyway, the patient was me, and the remedy worked!

A patient came to see me whose child had put her hand on an electric bar fire and had gone to hospital. The hospital had put the hand into a polythene bag full of bactericidal cream. So the mother was given *Arnica* 200c, the child was given *Arnica* 10M, and the child was also given *Causticum* 200c for the pain of the burns, and later *Calendula* 200c internally. I predicted that this hand would go septic as it was totally cut off from air, despite all that cream, a lot could happen. So I gave the mother *Pyrogenium* 10M to hold with detailed instructions, and advised her to keep in touch over the phone. I must have heard from them every day that week. That weekend sure enough she rang up and I asked had she called an ambulance? She said yes. Always call an ambulance, as any citizen could advise. I advised her to use the *Pyrogen*. She then called up saying my daughter is dancing! The little toddler was prancing about. I said, 'It is up to you to cancel the ambulance, but watch her if she needs two or three doses'. After that she came to my home, having at last agreed to take the polythene bag off, and I made gauze compresses of *Calendula* and showed her how to do that. What is very good, the only time it is useful, I think, is *Calendula* oil. The oil will enable the gauze not to stick. Circumcision is the only other time I use that.

I very rarely give only one dose in the mouth. It's likely to be two or three and to stop if there's a reaction. My experience is that people do things which they are not aware of, whether it is coffee, mint, perfume, mouthwash, cigarettes, things they take from other people whom they kiss. My experience goes back to my own career as a patient before I was even a proper student of homeopathy. Being given a remedy in a brown paper envelope, getting into the car and putting it into the side pocket. The car had just had a total rust treatment and it dawned on me, while in discussion with my homeopath, that that was probably why it did not work. I always dispense in glass and put the glass bottle into an envelope, if it is clear glass. Quite often patients are given three doses, and only take one or two, because of the instruction to stop if they get a reaction. After the first one, it is possible that nothing happened, but it is also possible that something did happen and if we had waited another week, its possible we might have noticed it. So this is an attempt to be practical.

**MS:** Have you ever had aggravations that have not gone on to amelioration at the end of it?

**FT:** Probably, although I do not have patients who have a lot of aggravations. There are people who have criticised me during intellectual discussion. They say, 'You do not have aggravations, you are not curing'. In Hering's original law it says that there has to be a skin eruption for cure to have taken place. So I am not sure whether one would call that an aggravation. Whatever the patient presents, from the inside out does mean skin eruption at the end, so that you have to see a skin eruption for cure to take place.

So if I have had aggravations, I think it might be the wrong remedy and re-take the case, just to be certain.

**MS:** How long would you wait?

**FT:** It's likely to be four weeks until the next consultation. Occasionally they ring up about the aggravation in about a week or two and I would say, 'Are you recovering', and they would say, 'Yes', and I would ask, 'Is it terrible to wait'? And if so, I'd tell them to have a coffee or brush their teeth. It does not seem to happen enough for me to put any emphasis on it.

**MS:** Do you actually always wait for a skin eruption at the end?

**FT:** It does not always happen. I would wait but the patients do not always hang about when they feel better.

**MS:** Do you have any enlightening information about sensitive patients and things that you have discovered that has not been documented before?

**FT:** Sniff. Ask the patient to sniff in one nostril and then the other. It has been pompously called 'olfaction'.

**MS:** Do you think that proves to be gentler?

**FT:** Yes.

**MS:** And if someone has a strong vitality, do you think they can take a higher potency?

**FT:** Yes, that certainly. If one has a higher vitality, then the higher the potency. In acutes, if they have a strong vitality. I have given a 200c to a gentleman of eighty-four with whooping cough, because he was a tough old man. He caught it from his grandchildren. Vithoulkas says, do not give homeopathy to people who have been on steroids for ten years. This gentleman had been on steroids for fifteen years and he had osteoporosis. The whooping cough got cured and he had less pain in his back.

**MS:** So if you have a hypersensitive patient are you likely to go down a bit or...?

**FT:** No, I am likely to think, sniff it! It is not the potency, it is them being sensitive. I do not see why a low potency is going to be any less aggravating to a sensitive patient if what they need is a high potency. Have you heard of a man called Kaspar Hauser?

He was a 19th century baby, born on the wrong side of the bedclothes to a nobleman and there was an inheritance problem. So they stuck him in a stable with the animals. He learned to eat on all fours, the case is documented in Clarke. When he finally emerged he was hypersensitive. He fell into the hands of the homeopaths. For him the story goes, 'The sound of wheat in the fields was like horses hooves. You only have to open the bottle in the room and he would get the remedy'. I do not know what it says about potency but in the end he received a dose of *Plumbum* at high velocity and he was assassinated because of this inheritance problem. A film was made about him called the *Enigma of Kaspar Hauser*.

**MS:** In terms of energy, I have been taught that one matches the energy of the person or the complaint with the energy in the remedy. And yet it's been my experience to have certain patients who have had for example psychotic episodes where the symptoms are incredibly vivid, and yet my gut feeling is that they are very sick and not to prescribe too high. I would imagine that perhaps this would be the same with someone having a heart attack, although I have never been in that situation. In terms of energy, what is happening there?

**FT:** I was once in a house that I owned, where in the basement there was a builder working. He was a beer drinker with a big belly, a middle aged chap and he had a heart attack. I gave him *Latrodectus mactans* 200c and he came around fantastically. He still went to hospital where he later died of complications but that initial attack was warded off very well with a 200c. Now if he had gone absolutely mad with his axe or his hammer, with a psychotic episode, if one could have got near him, I would have probably also given him a 200c. If I could not have got near him, I would have stuck it in water and hoped he would drink it.

200c is one I use in that sort of acute episode and I would not have wanted to go higher. Yes, you could have a psychotic aggravation and he could have gone even crazier.

**MS:** Do you have any questions that you would like answered?

**FT:** Yes, but I want to stick to the psychotic one here. I have only one that I can think of. I prescribed *Hydrogen* and it was for a man who had gone bonkers. What had happened was, he was sent to me by a rabbi. He was a Jewish man and had become a sort of born again Jew. He grew his beard six feet longer than mine, side locks, black hat, all the uniform, he was praying too hard, he was fasting too hard and he was trying to get himself at one with his maker. He was overdoing it and he had been sectioned. Basically he was psychotic and I gave him *Hydrogen* 1M. I did not know if it would have made him worse or better but it seemed the right remedy at the time. I do not often see people in a very psychotic state. It worked very well but the psychiatrist also went absolutely bonkers when he learned that the patient went off his normal medicine. Although the patient had actually calmed down, the psychiatrist did not look reality in the eye and they sectioned him again.

Questions I want answered. The physics of the micro-dose. There are many things to do with memory in water. There is a whole range of theories. What I am interested in is a historical thing. Do you know what afluxion potency is? Made by 19th century homeopaths, Skinner of Liverpool and Fincke and Swan of New York; Boericke & Tafel of Philadelphia had a Skinner fluxion potentiser. We take our potencies for granted. Succussion. The first variation of Hahnneman's idea of taking one drop out of a phial of which you have succussed and adding it to another bottle with ninety-nine drops of the liquid. It was Korsakov who tipped the liquid out, and used whatever was adhering to the bottle, and added ninety-nine drops of water which saves on bottles. But then there were men like Skinner of Liverpool and Fincke and Swan of New York, who developed machines where a high velocity of liquid was forced into a small vessel and what was left in the vessel was the potency. The physics of that seems to never have been investigated.

We now have modern machines. Quinn in San Rafael in California, Tony Pinkus of Ainsworths, John Morgan of Helios have all invented machines and Vithoulkas invented one which he used, but the Italian pharmacy went bust. These machines replicate the arm of a homeopath giving a wallop on a book. I think Hahnemann used the *Bible;* homeopaths now use the *Organon*. What is happening in succussion and are our potencies any different through using these different methods? There is an anthroposophical method of making the water go through a figure of eight trajectory with no shock, and I should love to know what that produces in the remedies.

How can we test a 10M from one place, and is it any different from a 10M from somewhere else? Is that why *drawer* homeopathy works?

# Roger Savage

**MS:** How do you choose a potency?

**RS:** It will depend on how broad and how deep the symptom picture is and also on the vitality of the patient.

**MS:** Could you be a little more specific with broad and deep?

**RS:** Are they suffering just one problem or several and how marked and severe is it and how deep rooted, how far back does it go, and how much of their being is it involving?

**MS:** And if all those things are true, and it's very deep and it has been going on for a long time etc, then would you choose a lower potency or a higher potency?

**RS:** I would expect a higher potency, unless the vitality was poor, in which case I would give a low potency and be content with possibly slower progress. I think we'd better establish if we're discussing centesimals!

**MS:** Well I was going to ask you, I presume you are talking about centesimals?

**RS:** Yes, because we just need to be sure that is what we are saying. And I will further fox you by saying that I presume we are talking about C3's. In other words, centesimals which have been triturated three steps.  I am very fond of the Q or LM potencies. But from the practicality point of view, if someone is not near a pharmacy for getting them or not near me for collecting it, I don't use them - it's practicality.

**MS:** What would make you choose an LM potency over and above a centesimal potency then?

**RS:** If a person had poor vitality or was extremely sensitive.

**MS:** Have you found that when using LM potencies, aggravations can happen?

**RS:** Oh yes, certainly.  But usually briefer and less severe.

**MS:** What would you do if someone phoned up and all hell is breaking loose and they were taking an LM daily?

**RS:** Well, they may get the effect from even one dose.  So if it has happened on a higher than LM1 then they need to change to having a dose of a lower potency. If it was a dose in a glass with a few drops from the bottle, they'll need to take another one, made with more steps of dilution from the original stock, because if one lowers or dilutes a potency, it does seem to act as a downward 'funnel' to reduce the aggravation from a dose.

**MS:** I have heard people doing that with centesimal potencies, but I have never heard of people doing that with LM's before, so that's really interesting.

**RS:** Same kind of principle.

**MS:** Do you always start with an LM1 or do you go higher generally?

**RS:** According to my sense of the patient.

**MS:** What would guide it?

**RS:** Sometimes a theoretical equivalent of LM and C3 potency. So, if I might give someone a 6c, I will use an LM1. If I might have given them a 12c, I could give them a LM3, if I might have given them a 30c, it would be a LM6.  If I might have given them a 200c, it would be an LM12.

**MS:** OK and how does that correspond?

194

**RS:** You have to multiply the Q or LM figures by 2.5, but it just was a perception of mine that those would be some energetic equivalents, even though the mathematics doesn't work out. 12 x 2.5 makes 30 rather than 200!

**MS:** And this has worked well for you?

**RS:** Yes, and it's not only if the centesimal was too powerful, but if the patient is the kind of patient who likes some back-up doses, then I don't want them to be repeatedly hit with a high centesimal. Those will be equivalent potencies that will just keep the hoop bowling along, so to say.

**MS:** Are you using C4[14] remedies?

**RS:** I would and I will but I haven't. Partly because I have only got very small stocks of a few C4 remedies and I would like to know a little bit more about the reported difference of picture that arises when you change the potency base. And yes, I don't want to start something that I can't follow through with.

But I am going to tell you something else startling about potencies, that not many of your interviewees will have said. I don't always use pharmacy potencies. There is nothing to beat a pharmacy potency, but the magnetic ones are a very good substitute and occasionally when pharmacies used to do their high potencies by older methods like high-pressure water jets, actually the magnetic ones sometimes seemed to be more accurate and more potent.

**MS:** How do you get a magnetic potency?

**RS:** I use what is called a Rae potentiser or simulator device. So that it's either a simulation which means it's derived from a card pattern, or it is a potency modification from a remedy sample.

**MS:** I won't ask you any more about that because it is a little bit too scientific for what I am trying to achieve here.

**RS:** The relevance is that one can produce in-between potencies easily or all kinds of variations readily. It means that I am not limited to 6c, 12c, 30c, 200c, 1M.

**MS:** What would make you choose an in-between potency?

---

[14] See interview with Alize Timmerman

**RS:** A sense that I wish to go just a little bit further than one of the standard ones, but not too much further. Now, I know that for many people a 12c is very physically active, maybe stirring, maybe jarring, so therefore I will prefer a 9c. If they are going along well on that but then run out of steam, I can go to a 15c which is gentle, and then an 18c, which has been found by some microscope research to dampen the activity of things like bacteria, so that is quite gentle. If I need to go by another step I can go to 24c, so working my way to 30c by easy steps. Now after 30c, I don't use 50c but I go to 60c, then 100c, then 200c. Now one person today has requested 300c, in other words wanting just a little whisker more. Often after 200c I go to 500c before a 1000c (1M). No pharmacy is stocking in-between potencies after 1000c, so that has to be magnetic, and 2M can be useful, 5M can be useful. Once in a rarity, I have gone from 10M to 20M before going to 50M, and certainly if in the almost unique moment one is working at the 100,000c (CM) level, and having to go further then obviously it's possible to go 200,000c then 500,000c (DM) before the 1,000,000c (MM). I cannot recall when I last had to go that high. I have a little suspicion that those sorts of potencies might well be needed in acute radiation sickness, where the vitality is good but the poisoning effects are severe and appalling, but we fortunately don't see that on a regular basis with the need to treat to that intensity.

**MS:** If you've found that a remedy hasn't worked, have you ever changed the potency and not the remedy?

**RS:** Yes.

**MS:** Have you done it successfully?

**RS:** Yes.

**MS:** When would you choose to do that? Presumably when you are sure of the remedy?

**RS:** Sure means reasonably sure and puzzled there is no response. I may then wonder if this patient is one of those people who tends to respond at higher levels. In other words, the active symptom roots are deep in the make up or deeply in the mental /emotional level. Some people, funnily enough, can be doing fantastically at 6c, 15c and so on. Others need 200c and higher before they show a reaction.

I have occasionally achieved cures at the level of 3c, 6c, 9c, and 15c for quite deep symptomatology. At the moment, for example, with candida symptoms, I have been giving potency LM1-LM4 and I sometimes use LMs like centesimals, in occasional doses.

**MS:** Right, you don't give a daily dose?

**RS:** Not always, because I know people have been trying this and finding that the action of a dose can last for quite some time. When I used the *Candida* remedy, even in centesimal, the 9c lasted for twelve months: now that to me is absolutely remarkable.

**MS:** Have you ever experienced aggravations in lower potencies and given higher potencies that have helped?

**RS:** In one particular case a patient had been given *Hepar sulph* 6c every two hours with no time limit! Not surprisingly he was doing badly, and was even developing sugar intolerance! I just had a hunch and gave *Hepar sulph* 1M. All the upheaval vanished within a day, but soon after the dose he felt a tremendous urging in the bowels, while on the underground and felt so anxious he took the train in the wrong direction. He only just got to a loo in time!!

**MS:** Do you usually descend the potency if there is an aggravation? Or wait?

**RS:** Yes, you can do it by ascending or descending, as I know by experience, but I am very cautious with the ascending method.

**MS:** Perhaps if you had tried and tested many times, you would feel better about it?

**RS:** Yes, having a sense though that high potencies are matching a very broad spectrum of a person, I'm wary of giving high if the malady is not covering the whole person, because I may distort their overall being.

I like to work up to those levels. I rather like the Jeremy Sherr view that the 100,000c (CM) is treating the whole tribe, the whole country. A recent homeopathy documentary pointed out that a 15c is a drop in the Atlantic and a 30c is a drop in all the oceans of the world. Well, for us the useful insight there, is just how potent even thirty steps makes it, and therefore a 10,000c (10M) is a drop in probably more than the solar system. They cannot understand what they have identified, but we should be very grateful for what they have just shown us.

**MS:** How far-ranging can something can be? Do you ever use prophylactics?

**RS:** Yes, if people are going on foreign holidays.

**MS:** In what potency or dosage do you tend to prescribe for that?

**RS:** I have a range of 30cs from Ainsworth.

**MS:** Do you prescribe them once a week?

**RS:** I have read, and haven't found it go wrong, that if they are going to have three or four such prophylactics, give one every two/ to three days until the range of requested nosodes has been covered and then repeat after about three or four weeks. Now I've no idea if I am doing any good, but to date no-one that has had that treatment has ever fallen foul of dreaded illnesses. I have known people, for example in India, who have taken nothing and then contracted typhoid for example.

**MS:** It's hard with prophylactics, because how do you know how long your remedies work for, there is nothing there to guide you, is there?

**RS:** Well, I know once when a 30c upset me - this was a *Staphysagria* - its period of action was about three months. I have just seen a couple who went to Thailand and they also wanted something for SARS. I think I gave them *Pneumococcinum* because I hadn't thought of *Oscillococcinum* at the time. Well they obviously didn't contract it. It's inexact, but it's also a helpful way of soothing patients' anxieties!

# Nancy Herrick

**MS:**   Can you tell me a little bit about how you decide upon which potency to use?

**NH:**   For me the remedy is the key. I don't put a lot of emphasis on potency, however I do have some ideas about it.

I use the clarity of the picture and I use the degree of the intensity of the illness. So, if the patient is quite ill and has a low vital force then I may use a very low potency. However, if they are quite ill and have a high vital force, like a little baby, I may use a very high potency like a 10M. If they are eighty-five and they have pneumonia I may use 6c. So, a lot of it does depend on the strength of the patient.

In a more typical case where they come in for more chronic symptoms, I often just use 200c or 30c. 200c is my most typical patient's first prescription. I usually keep the patient on the same remedy for years and years and years. And that's my ideal because then what happens, if it is really the right remedy, you just see that they get better and in a deeper and deeper way. I have also found that it takes many years to get into those bottom layers. For most people it's a really incredible process. I use the same remedy for acutes and that has really revolutionised my practice. I used to scramble for a new acute remedy every time they got some virus or whatever, now I don't do that at all.

**MS:**  Do you find that effective?

**NH:**  Very effective.  I used to get about ten phone calls a day on acutes and now I get very few because my patients know what to do. When they get something they just take their constitutional and they usually use 6c or 12c.  When I have a patient come in for the first time, I usually give them their high potency and I always give them a low potency to take home with them, usually it's a 12c or a 6c.  I tell them they can use that if they are getting sick; if they going to the dentist, if they are flying or if they have had a very stressful experience, or are about to have a very stressful experience.  I just tell them to take two pills of the 12c at their own discretion.  Then I say if you are getting sick, take that. You can take it two three days in a row, or, if you really are very stressed, you can take it every day for a short period. It tends to really help them.  It gives people something to do that works.

**MS:**  It sounds like that deals with the antidoting factor?

**NH:**  Sometimes it does and sometimes it doesn't.  Sometimes it's just not enough.  If they really antidote, they might need to go back to their 200c again.  Flying does interfere with remedies at times and so that can make a difference, taking the remedy before and after the flight.

**MS:**  Do you use ascending potencies, and go up the ascending scale as your patient's health starts to improve?

**NH:**  Yes I do.  Sometimes then I go down.

**MS:**  What would make you go down?

**NH:**  I stay with the same potency for as long as possible, just like Kent suggests.  Then, when that really isn't working anymore, I'll go up. However, if someone has done well for years and they come in with some minor symptoms, then I'll go down, and I'll just stay with the 30c; one dose of the 30c.

**MS:**  And that works well?

**NH:**  It does.

**MS:**  You spoke about the clarity of the picture and the degree and the intensity of the illness.  Do you find that they are almost the same thing; for example if somebody needs a high potency, the picture is very vivid?

**NH:** Well, sometimes the picture can be very vivid and not clear - we just don't know the remedy. Maybe I personally don't know the remedy because I have not studied enough or the remedy doesn't even exist.

**MS:** In terms of potency, what would you do in that instance?

**NH:** If I didn't know the remedy, or if I wasn't sure about the remedy, I would definitely go lower.

**MS:** What's your policy on aggravations?

**NH:** Actually my most common experience when seeing a patient is that I usually tell them to come back in a month, and they don't call me. So really, my most common experience is that they don't call me. They go through their aggravation, and sometimes I am amazed, they have had a horrendous time, but they often say, I just had a feeling that it was OK, or I just had this horrible headache for three days and I just went through it. Most of the patients that come here know about homeopathy and they've heard about it for years. They have been waiting for a long time to come and so they have some familiarity with it. They just have a certain amount of faith, I guess.

**MS:** My patients call me.

**NH:** Sometimes they call me of course, but mostly I don't hear from them. I hear about it at the follow up. If they call me I usually try to reassure them and don't give them anything to take. If I expect a potential severe aggravation like in an eczema condition I will warn the patient ahead and give them a very low potency like a 6c. By the way, I have not had the experience that LMs reduce the aggravation. Just the opposite in fact. I have seen horrendous aggravations from LMs.

**MS:** If a remedy does not work at all, have you ever changed the potency successfully, instead of changing the remedy?

**NH:** Yes, I have. I just had a case of a man who was going through extreme anxiety and I gave him *Silica*, his remedy is *Silica*. I knew his constitutional remedy as I've been treating him for fifteen years. So, I knew his remedy and it wasn't working, I had given him 10M and I even told him to take it three days in a row and it didn't work at all, so then I went to 50M, but I guess that's a different story from what you're asking. The 50M worked great. It worked within hours.

**MS:** It's not really a different story. You knew his remedy, but it can happen anyway. I have had quite a few cases like that and I have stuck to the remedy and it's worked for me.

**NH:** That's of course not always easy to do, to actually stick to the remedy. That's why I actually don't start out with really high potencies. I like to be able to work up.

**MS:** What are your views on dosage?

**NH:** What I always do is give one dose of the say 200c - half of a half gram bottle. They then keep half of a half gram bottle in storage somewhere, so if they get a relapse and call me, I can tell them to take the other half.

The other thing I do is use a creative approach to the potencies. I don't just go 30c, 200c, 1M, 10M, but Michael Quinn at our pharmacy will make any potency we want, so often, I do 30c, 200c, 1M and then I go to 2M or 5M, especially if I am really happy with the remedy and I don't want them to go up too fast. And that works great, because I can save those high potencies for when they really need it years later. I have patients on 5M for years. The other thing is, I use LMs a lot as boosters, so I'll put a person on 200c and then I'll put them on LM1, for people who are on drugs or medication.

**MS:** Will you do that at the same time?

**NH:** Yes. It's kind of unusual I know, but I like it very much. I just did that at our student clinic. A case of a young boy ten years old with chronic kidney failure. He was very ill. It was actually a case that was inappropriate for the student clinic. But it happened, and he was on ten different medications, including 60mg of Prednisone a day, which is extremely difficult. So, I put him on a 200c *Natrum sulphuricum*. Then I put him on LM1. Then I just automatically put him on to LM2 in a month, because he absolutely needed to be taking something every day and I am not happy with putting someone on 12c every day, because they need the change, they need to shift a bit. So I find LMs very useful for that. He has had a complete remission of his kidney failure and is doing very well emotionally as well.

**MS:** What would be your reason for giving the 200c first, to kick it all off or...?

**NH:** Yes, I also felt like he really needed something quite strong, to kick it off.

**MS:** Do you have any enlightening information to share with us about sensitivity and potency? You know, hypersensitive patients.

**NH:** I have been in practice almost thirty years and I have during that time had quite a few sensitives, what I call "the sensitives". Not a huge number, maybe twenty at the most, but these people are remarkable in that they just prove everything. Is that what you're talking about?

**MS:** Yes.

**NH:** They prove everything and they are incredible provers if you are doing a proving, but they are not very good homeopathic patients. When I feel I have someone who is truly a sensitive, I usually start out with flower essences just to see what happens. I will sometimes give one dose of a remedy, you know, one pill of a 6c, but often I start out with flower essences which are so gentle, and that is basically the only time I actually use them.

**MS:** Do you find that that helps in some way to strengthen up their vital force?

**NH:** Yes, I do, and they get a little more faith in you and they feel a little more trusting, and then very carefully you can start going into the real potencies. I have worked with those people and I am very careful in that way, and I've treated some of them quite successfully.

**MS:** The same sort of question about psychosis? Any enlightening information to share on psychosis and potency?

**NH:** I have cases that have done very well. I just had a young man of 22 years. The mother flew him in from across the country and I saw him. He was completely psychotic. I couldn't really get the case from him at all, it was "word salad". So, through talking to her I got the case. His remedy was very clear, it was *Veratrum album*. I gave him 10M. He was on medication of course so I gave it to him daily for five days. He was threatening people, he was quite violent, very suspicious. He was still doing very well six or eight months later, then I got a call and his father just decided spontaneously to give him a 10M since he had a cold. It really, really made him worse. He completely relapsed. So then I just said wait and he did come out of it.

That's the other thing I would like to say that is fairly important, there are a lot of people out there who are giving remedies in high potencies indiscriminately. I can tell you from my years of experience you can really create havoc in a case that way. I mean most of us know that, but there are some homeopaths teaching that and it is really scary to see that. I have done it myself. I have mistakenly given someone a high potency again when they are doing well and they are just coming in complaining about minor things and they have a terrible reaction. To think that homeopaths are doing that as their regular practice is very disturbing.

**MS:** OK, so if you clearly see the picture then go high even in psychosis.

**NH:** In that instance the picture was very clear, although I was still a little nervous about it, but that is what I did, 10M for five days. He was such an extreme case. He was mentally very ill but physically very healthy and so I thought I should go in very high.

**MS:** And finally hyperactivity, how would that sway your choice of potency?

**NH:** I would go high, and unless they are on medication I won't repeat it. The repeated high potency is usually for people on medication or sometimes really extreme mental illness requires repeated high potencies. Usually, even if the picture is clear, I won't repeat the high potency without seeing them, or talking to them.

# Jeremy Sherr

**(It is Jeremy's special request that I spell homeopathy as homoeopathy in this interview)**

**MS:** Can you tell me a bit about how your potency selection has evolved over the years?

**JS:** When it comes to potency there are three avenues of knowledge, and these are the three main avenues of study in homoeopathy; cases, materia medica and philosophy. This is the triangle that makes up all homoeopathic study and knowledge. So, in my investigation of looking for ways to choose the optimal potency for the case, I took the approach of studying via the above three avenues.

I will begin by explaining my approach via cases. My technique for learning from cases was to use a single potency for a long time. When I began practice and wanted to have a feeling for the potencies, I prescribed only the 30c potency for my first year. In my second year of practice, I prescribed mainly 200c and the occasional 30C, and for my third year I prescribed mainly 1M, and only occasional 30c and 200c. Only after that did I go on to 10M and using the whole range of potencies. So, by concentrating on one potency for a whole year I got a feeling for what each potency is capable of doing. That was my approach to learning about potency via cases.

**MS:** What did you learn about the 30c, 200c, IM, etc?

**JS:** I learnt that how potencies act is in relationship to the person they are given to, not the simple idea of this potency does one thing and another does something else.

I was surprised how potent the 30c is and how long it lasts. That was my main feeling. There were cases where I gave one dose of a 30c and it will last two months, six months or even one year. I realised that the 30c was quite powerful and long-acting and could touch most pathologies. As to the 200c, there is a myth that goes around that it is a very active and dangerous, a hyperactive potency. I can't say that I find that in my experience, but it may be more intense than the 30c. In terms of length of action I cannot say that it lasts longer. It depends on which potency the patient needs.

Trying to assign certain characteristics to certain potencies can be very deceptive. The length and depth of action of a remedy is a result of degree of similarity, as well as the nature of the remedy, so that comparing potency action between different cases or remedies is misleading. It is also often the case that less similar remedies work better in lower potencies, while more similar ones work all the way to the top.

What is more significant is the nature of the jump between potencies in one case, i.e. from a 30c to a 200c, from a 200c to a 1M, from a 1M, to a 10M. For instance, in my experience, the jump from 200c to 1M is not as powerful as the jump from 30c to 200c.

**MS:** How does materia medica influence your potency choice?

**JS:** My second avenue of approach is through materia medica and the primary investigation of the materia medica is through provings. The principle of homoeopathy, like cures like, means we find out what remedies can cure from doing a proving. Why not apply the same rule to potency? Essentially, that is the most logical way to approach potency, by finding out in a proving what a potency can do. So, seeing to date I have done twenty-five Hahnemannian provings and used a variety of potencies in these provings, I have also found out various things about them. In fact, at one stage I used to put all these provings into a database, so that I could analyse the potencies relative to the symptoms they produced. Ultimately, this approach means that if we were really precise in homoeopathy, we would match the potency to the potency that produced the symptom in the proving. For example, if a person suffered from a left-sided migraine at 6am and we found a suitable remedy, we could look up the potency that produced this symptom, according to the law of similars. In order to do that we need a database because it's too difficult to look up the symptom and potency every time. So, if Allen's Encyclopaedia was databased, or if the computer repertories could attach the original potency that produced the symptom, we would approach a stage where it is quite possible to find the potency which produced it, like curing like.

One thing I can definitely say from both the cases and the provings is that the notion that high potencies affect the mentals and low potencies affect the physicals is inaccurate. That's my opinion derived from many provings. In provings, some of the strongest mental/emotional symptoms have come from a 6c and yet with a 200c I have occasionally seen none of the mental/emotionals but more physicals, and also vice versa, which means that the mental/emotional/physical hierarchy does not apply to potency. In fact, to my mind, it does not apply to much at all. I have had cases that are mental/emotional cases which have been greatly helped with low potencies; LM1s, LM2s, 6cs, 12cs and I have seen the opposite in terms of higher potencies and physical conditions. I have seen provings from a single dose of 12c last for months. These facts contradict some of the prevailing notions on the subject.

**MS:** What about the philosophical approach?

**JS:** To me, philosophy is the most important of the three, because that is the source and reason behind what we do. If there is no philosophy, the clinic and the materia medica will just go round in circles without true direction.

You are not going to find the philosophy of potency in the *Organon*, there are no precise rules on what potency will treat. In fact, there is some confusion in the *Organon* in this regard, and this is because of the confusion between dose and potency which are often interchangeable, so that one does not know if dose means the quantity of the medicine, two granules, four granules etc. or the potency of the medicine. Usually, it seems to actually mean a mixture of both, so it is very difficult to decide on potency according to Hahnnemann's instruction.

In relation to potency selection I refer to paragraph 16 in the *Organon*. I have published a summary of my thoughts about that paragraph in my book on Syphilis. I don't go deeply into potency selection there, but it is an introduction to my opinion on this issue. Paragraph 16 says "a dynamic disease can only be caused by a dynamic pathogen". So what is a dynamic pathogen, and what does dynamic mean? Dynamic means capable of motion, something that moves, that lives. So, if the vital force is something that moves and is capable of change, it can only be affected dynamically by something that moves and is capable of change. That is Hahnemann's first premise in paragraph 16. His second premise in this paragraph is that if diseases are dynamic then they can only be affected by dynamic remedies, meaning remedies that are capable of change and movement. This is the reason we dynamise our remedies, put motion into them. That is Hahnemann's logical equation: disease is dynamic, vital force is dynamic, and therefore we need dynamic remedies.

From this I concluded that we should be able to measure the dynamis of a remedy according to the dynamic level of disease that the person has. Meaning, we need to match the potency of the remedy to the disease. This is why I think there is a lot of confusion in the subject of potency, because most people discuss what is a 30c, what is a 200c, what is a 1M, but I don't think they are measurable entities on their own. What matters is the nature of the interaction between potency and the diseased person. So the 10M for one person is not a 10M for another person and therefore in my opinion generalising is impossible.

For this reason I set about finding a way of measuring the dynamic level of each person and their disease and matching it to the various dynamisations, and creating a system by which we can match one to the other in regards to similar levels of dynamis. By levels of dynamis I mean the following: a person in health is at their most dynamic, capable of a full range of motion, capable of change. They have one hundred percent response ability in every direction, can adapt to any situation, they have total freedom of action. Now a person in disease is a person who becomes more and more static and restricted, not capable of motion, change or adaptation. A person who is dead has zero dynamis and therefore is not capable of any adaptation, change or motion.

To measure these levels I have created a scale of dynamis to static ranging from ten to zero. Ten is a totally healthy person, with maximum dynamic factor; zero is a dead person who is totally static and incapable of change or adaptation. I developed criteria for measuring the level of dynamic/stuckness in a person, a way of defining precisely what is a nine, a six and a three. I will not go into details here as this is a lengthy subject and beyond the scope of this interview, but once learnt it is easy to apply. My students know it by the abbreviation MOPMECS, namely Modalities, Obstacles, Pathology, Mentals, Energy, Creativity and Sensitivity.

In a similar way, potencies can also be defined from the most static, mother tincture (zero), to the totally dynamised MM (ten). Using this system I match the static/dynamic level of disease to the static/dynamic level of potency. The results have been very pleasing. I have been teaching this system for fifteen years and the feedback that I get from the students is excellent, in terms of helping them to find a suitable potency and in terms of results.

**MS:** Therefore if somebody is at their most healthy, they get a higher potency?

**JS:** Correct, if somebody is at their most healthy, they will need a higher potency and less dose. For example, a person is very healthy except that they get a sore throat once a year on a certain day, let's say on a blue moon, and other than that they adapt easily to every situation. They are very dynamic and need a highly potentised remedy which is very dynamic like them. Like cures like in potency. But a person with cancer, schizophrenia, arthritis or any other very stuck disease, is going to need a very static potency. That is why Cooper used the (arborivital) mother tincture to cure cancer very successfully.

Another ramification of this idea is that acute diseases, which are by nature more dynamic, will respond better to higher potencies. We have certainly seen fevers that have been promptly cured by the 50M, where the same remedy in 30C did very little.

**MS:** You mentioned jumping from 30c to the 200c, from the 200c to the 1M, that you have some interesting information there.

**JS:** People try to generalise regarding each potency, but this is difficult as we are prescribing for people with different dynamic levels. You may have a 10M lasting three days in one person, and in another person a 30c lasts two years. How potencies act is in relationship to the person they are given to, not the simple idea of this potency does one thing and the other does something else. But you can judge potencies in relation to the same patient's progression. When you have exhausted a particular potency and you go up to the next potency, then you can see the relative difference of strength between the two. So for instance a jump from a 30c to a 200c is usually quite a good jump and usually carries on and continues the good results, but I have found that a 200c to a 1M is often not substantial enough. Even from the purely mathematical point of view, it's not a significant jump. That is why some people think that the 1M is a weak potency, but they wouldn't think it was weak as a first potency. This scale, 12C, 30C, 200C 1M, 10M, 50M etc comes from Kent, it is what he found empirically. These are very arbitrary numbers. You could wonder why he chose 1M not the 2.5. Also, Kent used a different kind of potency. Some of them were hand-made in a variety of methods that were possibly more (or less) powerful.

**MS:**   I wonder why he chose the standard potencies we use?

**JS:**   I think it was an arbitrary choice based on convenience rather then a precise series. It's really too neat to be relating to a real natural series. Perhaps a Fibonacci series[15] would be more appropriate.   I find the 200c to the 1M is not always a good jump, the 1M to the 10M is okay, but the 10M to the 50M is weak. You can start a case with a 50M with good effect, but I have often found that when I exhaust the 10M and go up to a 50M, it is often not a sufficient jump.

**MS:**   So then what do you do?  Do you to up to a CM?

**JS:**   You go up to a CM, or an MM, or down to a 12c or 30c.

**MS:**   Using your way of prescribing potency, what is your experience with aggravations?

**JS:**   Though I see a few aggravations, my experience is that using my method of choosing potency does minimise them. Generally I do like a short harmless aggravation!  Kent says that the homoeopath prefers a cure with some aggravation. Obviously I don't relish severe bothersome or prolonged aggravations.  If that does happen, it is often due to a poorly chosen potency.

**MS:**   If you have a case where you have a bad aggravation and your chosen potency has not been so great in your own mind, do you use another potency to try and correct that?

---

[15] The infinite sequence of numbers in which each number is the sum of the previous two. *Collings English Dictionary*

**JS:** I usually try and wait through it. If it is really severe, I might go to a vastly different potency to try and reduce the problem, but I do this very rarely. For instance, if I have given a 10M, I might later try giving a dose of a 12c or an LM. I find that moving down from a 10M to 30c or 12c is often very useful and I go down as freely as I go up.

In the old days, a high potency used to be considered as a gentle prescription. These days, people consider a high potency as an aggressive dangerous potency. In the old days homoeopaths often thought, I'd better be careful, I'll give a 50M. Nowadays, people think I'd better be careful, I'll give a 30c. And the truth is that both are right because it depends on the case and not the potency.

**MS:** Do you ever go up in potency if you have a bad aggravation?

**JS:** Usually I go down.

**MS:** Would you ever choose to change the remedy due to an aggravation?

**JS:** Very rarely. I don't like to do that. Certainly not while the remedy is acting, unless it is a situation where many new and troublesome symptoms develop, in which case it is a bad proving and should be antidoted at once (see *Organon* paragraph 249).

**MS:** If a remedy hasn't noticeably shifted anything at all within a reasonable time frame, have you ever changed the potency and not the remedy successfully?

**JS:** Occasionally. I think it can happen in approximately 5% of cases, not often. I have often questioned my classes on this, and out of all the homoeopaths I have asked, probably over a thousand, about 3-5% of the students have changed potency in a case with good effect when the remedy has not worked previously. And these cases would be one out of many cases that each of these homoeopaths see. So it can happen, but not often.

On the other hand, bear in mind that many homoeopaths never try changing the potency, so that this statistic may be inaccurate. So I would recommend trying the remedy in a different potency if you are either very confident of the remedy or have seen a slight action of the remedy.

**MS:** What are your views on dosage?

**JS:** I read a correspondence between Boenninghausen and Hahnemann in which they agreed that eight poppy seeds was too much, so they had gone down to giving two poppy seeds. Since then I have gone down to giving one or two tablets only and I found that to be fine. I have had occasional experience with patients who mistakenly took too many tablets and had bad aggravations as a result. I remember a case where a patient got a bottle of LM poppy seeds, one of which was meant to be diluted in the stock bottle, but they misunderstood and took a whole teaspoon, and had a horrendous aggravation. So, I tend to send people two tablets: one to take and one to drop on the carpet.

**MS:** When do you choose to use water remedies?

**JS:** I do use water remedies a lot, either in centesimal form or in LM form but especially in acutes that are anything less than mild. Any acute that is going to be prolonged, pneumonia, bronchitis, etc., I'll use a water remedy, which I find more effective.

**MS:** Do you have any enlightening information relating to potency in the following three cases; the first one is hypersensitive people?

**JS:** Hypersensitive people can be a homoeopath's nightmare. Kent says that you should stick to a 30c or 200c. I tend to find that this is too high. What I usually do is take a dose of 12c, put it in a litre bottle of water, shake it up and give them one teaspoon of that, or put one teaspoon of the resulting solution into another litre bottle of water and give them one teaspoon of that.

**MS:** The second one is psychosis?

**JS:** I view that as a very stuck condition and will therefore use a low potency or LM, repeated.

**MS:** And hyperactivity?

**JS:** I view hyperactivity as a stuck disease, although superficially it seems to be energetic. It is a false dynamis which is really static, stuck on activity. I therefore tend to use lower potency, repeated. When I say repeated in all these cases, I mean repeated as long as there is improvement, but stop with any aggravation. However I do consider all the parameters, so a healthier child with some hyperactivity will get a higher potency.

**MS:** Do you have any useful anecdotes that have changed your views about potency or dosage in a big way?

**JS:** In terms of dosage, I worked for two years giving the remedy mainly by olfaction, a single sniff from the bottle. So I know what olfaction can do, which may seem less than a material dose but usually acts more powerfully. It is very interesting to observe the immediate reaction after a remedy by olfaction. From this and other experience I have learnt that, in terms of dosage, less is more.

**MS:** Why did you abandon it?

**JS:** I didn't. I did it for two years and I learnt a lot and now I use it occasionally when the circumstances are right. Patients can get a bit sceptical, they need something material to take. Also, the immediate action is often much more powerful, to the degree that I have seen people faint on the spot after a sniff, so when I use it I make sure they can relax for 15 minutes after.

**MS:** When you give a remedy these days by olfaction, what are your reasons for doing so?

**JS:** If I want to see a quick action, or if I want to observe the reaction to the remedy in the clinic. Those would be the two main reasons. Occasionally some patients are anxious about taking the pills. It's amazing how people will swallow ten kilos of antibiotics and steroids, but when you want to give them one little pill they become petrified. In those cases it might be easier for them to receive a dose by olfaction.

**MS:** Do you make them sniff the pills or the liquid?

**JS:** The pills are fine, Hahnemann used them too. Another interesting thing Hahnemannn describes in the end of *The Chronic Diseases* is how to apply liquid potencies directly to the body. I have tried it a few times and the results have been good. It is a useful addition, especially for people who want to be doing something 'practical'. Hahnemann was very enthusiastic about this method, he felt it speeded up the cure greatly.

**MS:** Tell me about LMs.

**JS:** I use LMs in 40% of my practice. I use them any time that I find that the stuckness on my scale is lower than a four or five out of ten, especially in any case where there are obstacles to cure. The one thing I find about LMs is that when they have had the remedy for more than a month, it's better to jump two levels up, i.e. from the LM1 to LM3 and LM3 to LM5, rather than just raising one potency at a time. This is because they often passed the level of the next potency by continually succussing for two or more months.

Another thing is that many homoeopaths always start with LM1, but there is no logical reason for this, it is just a fixed idea. Just as we don't start every case with a 12C, we shouldn't always start with LM1. It is a very low potency really. I start with any LM, according to what is appropriate to the case, though I must say that over LM10 is quite high and should be reserved for dynamic patients. There is also an art to choosing even or odd LMs, I find that one scale suits some patients better then others.

**MS:** What would make you decide to start on a higher LM?

**JS:** The level of stuckness. The more dynamic the case the higher I will go. So if you have very stuck case, say a level 2/10 on my scale, and you start with a LM 18, you may get a big aggravation. On the other hand I've had patients with cancer who started with a LM1 and did very well, and after five years they are on LM53, still doing well. This works very well when appropriate, whereas if I started them on such a high potency I think they would have suffered. There is a big difference between the initial potency and the follow-up potency.

LM's can aggravate horrendously. But the aggravation often comes after a month or two, when they have had enough of the remedy, so that it should be stopped for a week or ten days before going up a level or two. It is also important to give every patient a break from the LM once in a while, otherwise you will never see the rebound or relapse, which is an important indicator.

**MS:** Do you have any questions that you would like answered on potency?

**JS:** A prover of *Neon*, which is a very mathematical remedy, states that we need to be extremely precise about potency, even to the difference between the 6c and 7c. But at this time no one knows how to be that exact. Within the next ten or twenty years somebody may invent a machine that can measure potency fields and vibrations, a machine that can also measure people's dynamic vital force electronically, and then we will be able to really know the precise potency for each person. Until then we can only use the crude methods we have been talking about. What I would like to know is if *Arnica* 200c is the same as *Calcarea carbonica* 200c? Is a mineral 30c the same as an animal 30c? Because if it is not, then even trying to compare the 200c of one remedy with the 200c of another is a waste of time. If potency differs from remedy to remedy then the whole issue is much more complicated. At this time we can only make rough assessments, but these should include the source of the remedy, its physical dose, and the state of the patient. So there is much to learn.

# Alize Timmerman

**MS:**   How do you choose a potency, what method do you use?

**AT:**   It relates to the pathology of the patient.

**MS:**   Can you be a little more specific?

**AT:**   I use a lot of C4 potencies, which are made differently and I will explain that to you later on.  I choose the 12 C4, but when the case is on an emotional level, then I choose 30 C4 and when the centre of focus is more mental/emotional I choose a 1300 C4.  If the patient needs help spiritually then I choose the highest of the C4 remedies.

**MS:**   Do you ever use C3 potencies anymore?

**AT:**   Yes, I use them very often, but they do not work on the highest level. That is very clear.

**MS:**   So in your experience, the remedies that I use, the C3 remedies, are less efficient?

**AT:**   Yes.

**MS:** I was at the Society of Homeopaths conference in Keele a few years ago when I first learnt of these different triturations of remedies and I guess that this would be a good time for me to ask you more about them and what you do to achieve these potencies. How do you make them?

**AT:** I can send you an exact procedure[16]. The normal remedies you use are triturated as Hahnneman writes in the *The Chronic Diseases* up to C3 trituration, and with the C4 we only triturate one or sometimes two steps more.

**MS:** On the pathological level as well, do you feel your remedies are more efficient?

**AT:** Yes, but especially when the pathology comes from the spiritual plane in deep diseases, like cancer. For example, the breast is the material plane and in its pathology it is expressed on the physical level, but it comes from the spiritual level.

**MS:** Cancer is traditionally very difficult for homeopaths to treat.

**AT:** Exactly, so I came to this understanding through better results with C4 potencies.

**MS:** Do we have them in England?

**AT:** No, but you can buy them in Germany and I can send you the address.[17]

**MS:** What I usually ask people is, does your choice of potency ever let you down, but I know, because I was at that conference, that your choice of potency did let you down one time when you were certain of the remedy and that was how you were inspired to discover these C4 triturations. Do you find that if you have given what I would call an ordinary centesimal potency, or in other words a C3, and you are sure of the remedy and it hasn't worked, and then you use a C4, it then works?

**AT:** Very well. Yes, that is how I came to this. With many of my cases that did not go well, or let's say the patient did well for a certain while, for a year or something, and then the result wasn't there anymore. But when I started to use the C4 potencies with these patients, I had very good results again.

---

[16] Refer to website, www.hahnemanninstuut.nl

[17] Refer to website, www.hahnemanninstuut.nl

**MS:** Is there any instance where you would think that the C3 remedies are better?  More efficient?

**AT:** I've been in practice for 22 years, so I have had many good results with C3 remedies also, but the C4s are an addition.  You see, we had many steps with the C3 potencies and this adds something.  It's not something new but rather a development that comes after the C3 remedies.

**MS:** Do you start off with the C4s or with the C3s?

**AT:** I use to start with the C3s but in the last year I now start off with the C4s.

**MS:** What about aggravations  with these new potencies?

**AT:** You don't see so many aggravations with these potencies because they work much more on the spiritual level, so there is not much aggravation on the physical level.  What I mean by spiritual level is that the patient has more questions around what their purpose is, what goal they want to follow, or they do not know their purpose.  These kind of life questions or existential questions are part of the C4 level.  If you give a remedy on that level, you can also give a remedy on the lower level in a C3 potency, and you can give them together.

**MS:** Can you tell me a little more about giving remedies together in that way?

**AS:** I have not done it that often, but I've done it in deep problematic cases.  For example, in an acute you can prescribe a  remedy in C3 potency and it can go together with a remedy that is prescribed more on a C4 level.

**MS:** So, would you give a chronic remedy when you saw the patient and if they had an acute, an interim acute, you could actually use an ordinary C3 remedy?

**AT:** Or an LM potency.

**MS:** One of the questions I have been asking all the homeopaths that I have spoken to is what they do if a patient does aggravate? Some homeopaths tend to treat an aggravation while others don't.

**AS:** In the first place I just wait.  If the aggravation takes too much of the vital force, what you can easily do is take the same remedy, dissolve it in 30ml of water and shake it a few times and take six drops out of it then dissolve those six drops in some water and give it to the patient for three days. In this way you can take away the aggravation.

**MS:** And would you use the 30c potency even if you had already given the 30c potency, for example?

**AT:** Yes, you can do it with the same potency. But, if you are not confident about it, then take a lower one of the same remedy.

**MS:** Have you ever used a higher potency to make a remedy more gentle?

**AT:** No. I haven't had many aggravations, so in my own opinion, it gets too much attention, because it's not normal practice and it makes people scared. Even the word is not right, I would like to say a reaction. A reaction from the remedy is better. Aggravation is a negative kind of explanation, which is not at all what is happening to the patient. A reaction to the body from the action of the remedy is a much better way of saying it.

**MS:** Yes, you are right the word has a negative connotation! What are your views on dosage?

**AT:** I often give the patient three doses in three days with 24 hours in between. If there is a reaction they stop taking the remedy. With C4 remedies, I usually give them only once. I use LM potencies when the patient is in a very slow kind of process and for a period of 21 days, I tell the patient to take ond dose a day, then stop for a week then call me to talk about how they proceed.

**MS:** So something very slow may be something perhaps like arthritis that someone has had for many years?

**AT:** Yes.

**MS:** When you repeat a curative remedy, what makes you change the potency?

**AT:** When the patient is getting better I don't do anything. When the patient is a little bit worse I repeat the remedy, and when the same remedy does not do anything anymore then I give a higher potency, but I can also choose a lower potency.

**MS:** What would make you choose a lower potency?

**AT:** When I have the feeling that the potency that I've given is not working too well and when the patient is not strong.

**MS:** So if the remedy is not working so well, and has done previously, and the patient is strong then you would go up in potency.

**AT:** Yes.

**MS:** Are there any other situations apart from slow processes that would make you choose a water potency, an LM for example?

**AT:** Yes, in older people and in people who want to take a remedy every day. With LM potencies you have a better possibility to regulate a reaction. With the C potencies you can have strong reactions while with LM you have softer reactions.

**MS:** I have used LMs quite a lot and I have found that sometimes the reaction one can sometimes get from an LM can be just as strong as from a C potency.

**AT:** So then you have to dissolve it in a second or a third glass. So we have to dilute it a little bit more.

**MS:** Apart from aggravations would you plus remedies for any other reason?

**AT:** Now and then I have used the system of Ramakrishnan. Very seldom, but I have sometimes given my patients repeated very soft doses. In cancer, you can have very strong reactions and that is not right when the disease process is so extreme that the healing force of the body cannot follow.

**MS:** Do you find that your C4 remedies are gentler?

**AT:** I cannot say that because they work on a different level.

**MS:** But you find that if you put a remedy in water, then it makes it more gentle in terms of reactions?

**AT:** I cannot confirm that, because I have seen many different reactions.

**MS:** Do you have any information to share with us as far as maintaining causes are concerned?

**AT:** I think we have to give more doses sometimes, but it then becomes very clinical homeopathy, and it can become like suppression, but then maybe we have to suppress sometimes. You know that's part of our work also and sometimes there is no choice.

**MS:** Do you have any insight into treating very sensitive people, hypersensitive people?

**AT:** We should try using the C4 potencies, the higher potencies, on them. I haven't tried it but I would like to see what happens when we do.

**MS:** My final question is do you have any questions on potency and dosage that you personally would like answered?

**AT:** I would like others to tell their experiences of giving a remedy in two different potencies at the same time. I think there are a lot of questions around this.

# ACKNOWLEDGEMENTS

Jon Shine for your love, support, caring and huge input. Matt, Becca and Dan for being in the world. Elaine and David Ratner; my parents for being the wonderful parents that they are. Thalia Vines and Karen Hirsch, the first people I phoned; you helped me get the ball rolling. Rajan Sankaran, whose inspiration is now indelibly woven into the tapestry of my work. Lilya Pasea and Cher Strydom for transcribing the taped interviews. Nick Churchill, Miranda Castro, Arlene Cohen, Lesley Becker, Jon Shine, Rowena Ronson and Norman Shine for your hours of hard work proof reading and editing, and making this a better book. Ruth Kaye for your graphic art; you have the Midas touch. David Witko, Ruth, and Barbara at Miccant, thank you for your contribution, your help and for putting up with me. Margreet at Links magazine. All my interviewees and a special thank you to Miranda Castro; I feel honoured, what can I say? Cassandra Marks, my homeopath, for keeping me well; I am not an easy patient. Sylvia Prescott, my amazing yoga teacher (I could not be a homeopath if I did not practice yoga).

# Useful Addresses

John Morgan,
Helios Pharmacy Ltd.,
89-97 Camden Road,
Tunbridge Wells,
Kent,
TN1 2QR.
Tel: 01892 537254
Email: www.retail@helios.co.uk

David Witko (Isis),
Miccant Ltd.,
14, Mulberry Close,
West Bridgford,
Nottingham,
NG2 7SS.
Tel: 0870 141 7053
Email: micant@micant.com

Mike Bridger,
Contemporary College of Homeopathy,
Exeter,
Devon.
Tel: 01626 873903

Orion Advanced Training in Homeopathy,
Tel: 0207 624 8650 & 01626 873 903

Francis Treuherz,
The Homeopathy Helpline.
Tel: 09065 343404
Website: www.homeopathyhelpline.com

Rowena Ronson,
Homeopathic Support Group,
North London/Hertfordshire.
Tel: 0208 386 2170.

Roger Savage,
Rae Machines,
26, Winstanley Road,
Saffron Walden,
Essex,
CB11 3EQ.
Tel: 01799 524442
Mobile: 07889 989398

Ian Watson,
The Lakeland College,
Postal Buildings.
Ash Street,
Bowness–on-Windermere,
Cumbria. LA23 3EB.
Tel: 01539 447666
Fax:

Jeremy Sherr,
The Dynamis School,
39 Wells Road,
Malvern,
WR14 4RJ
Webstite: www.dynamis.edu

I consider this book to be a work in progress and would like to invite my readers to send cases that highlight useful new discoveries about potency and dosage.

It is my intention to one day update the information contained herein.


My address:

Room 6,
Concorde House,
Grenville Place,
Mill Hill,
London,
NW7 3SA.